STEP-BY-STEP
YOGA
for Conception, Pregnancy, Birth and Beyond

FRANÇOISE BARBIRA FREEDMAN
AND DORIEL HALL

LORENZ BOOKS

For Joanna and all babies who have a tough start, yet smile through life

This edition is published by Lorenz Books, an imprint of Anness Publishing Ltd,
108 Great Russell Street, London WC1B 3NA; info@anness.com

www.lorenzbooks.com; www.annesspublishing.com

If you like the images in this book and would like to investigate using them for publishing,
promotions or advertising, please visit our website www.practicalpictures.com for more information.

© Anness Publishing Ltd 2014

A CIP catalogue record for this book is available from the British Library.

Publisher: **Joanna Lorenz**
Additional text: **Doriel Hall**
Project Editors: **Debra Mayhew, Ann Kay**
Designer: **Lisa Tai**
Jacket design: **Adelle Mahoney**
Photographers: **Alistair Hughes and Christine Hanscombe**
Stylist: **Sue Duckworth**
Illustrator: **Samantha Elmhurst**

PUBLISHER'S NOTE
The reader should not regard the recommendations, ideas and techniques expressed and described
in this book as substitutes for the advice of a qualified medical practitioner or other qualified
professional. Any use to which the recommendations, ideas and techniques are put is at the
reader's sole discretion and risk.

Contents

introducing
yoga

Yoga is a holistic life practice that
will greatly help you to enjoy your
pregnancy, right from conception
through to the birth, and beyond.
The specially adapted exercises in this
book are easy to follow, and a pleasure
to perform, whether or not you have
ever done yoga before. They will
increase your vitality, reduce your stress
levels and make you feel close to your
growing baby long before he or she is
born as well as in the first few months.

How yoga works for you

Yoga is a holistic discipline so it benefits you at every level, not only the physical one. Yoga philosophy maintains that a human being operates at several well-defined levels.

the five levels

There are five principal levels in yoga, and these are as follows.

Physical structure This includes bones, joints, muscles, skin and internal organs. Yoga develops physical strength, stamina and suppleness but these qualities are also developed at mental and emotional levels. Movement and posture are key elements.

Life processes This is the working of all the bodily systems, such as the respiratory and

cardiovascular systems, the various branches of the nervous system, the hormonal system, the digestive system and, of course, the reproductive system that will first create your baby and then support it in the womb. Breathing is the key element.

Internal organization This governs the workings of the brain and nervous system, so that all other body systems get the energy they need to do their jobs, just when they need it. In this way, internal harmony (also known as homeostasis) is sustained and we enjoy a state of contented well-being. Relaxation is the key element.

Clarity of mind This involves the ability to sort out our priorities, to concentrate on just one subject at a time until we are ready to turn our attention to another, rather than being too easily distracted by conflicting demands. In this way, we use our energy in a focused fashion, alternating periods of activity with those of relaxation. Being aware of posture, breathing and relaxation, and bringing them together in yoga practice, is a form of meditation, and meditation is a key element here.

△ Take time to relax and commune with your baby. This Walking Meditation (29) will help you to focus on the most important things in your life.

△ Yogic stretching, relaxing and unwinding with your partner helps you open up to each other.

Emotions and deepest desires Yoga differentiates between automatic reactions and considered responses. We choose to respond warmly and positively to life rather than spin from one knee-jerk reaction to another. In this way, we take control of our lives and cultivate qualities of the heart. We develop mental stamina, plus emotional as well as physical suppleness and strength. Taking time and trouble to make a resolution that is meaningful for us, and confirming it while in deep relaxation, helps us to live more fully as the person that we choose to be – truly living our choices.

the Chakras

In simple terms, the Chakras are the points where the five levels of being, already described, meet and work together to produce the person that we are. The Chakras correspond to nerve plexuses along the spine in the physical body, and yoga aims to bring them into balance with each other in order to keep us healthy, happy and growing in wisdom and serenity.

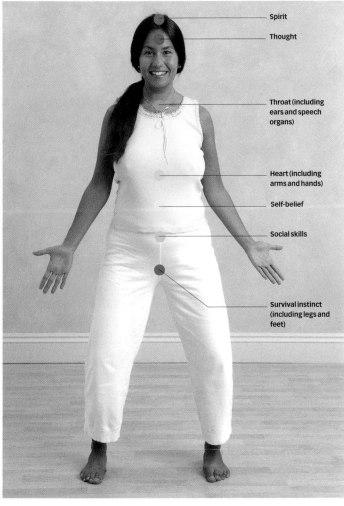

Spirit

Thought

Throat (including ears and speech organs)

Heart (including arms and hands)

Self-belief

Social skills

Survival instinct (including legs and feet)

◁ The position of the Chakras in the human body. These fall into three main areas: the Life area (waist to toes), the Love area (chest and throat), and the Light area (head).

Love energies The two Chakras in the chest area are concerned with relationship, or Love energies. The heart is often called the "organ of feeling", and we express those feelings through the voice box in the throat. How we breathe profoundly influences our nervous system, which in turn determines to a large extent how we are feeling in ourselves and towards other people. Breathing with awareness could be said to be the heart of yoga, as all the other practices are linked with the movements of our breath. Relaxed breathing and deep relaxation practices allow us to open our hearts in welcome to all those beings we interact with, as well as to ourselves.

Light energies The two Chakras in the head are concerned with our mental, or Light, energies. It is these that sustain the clarity of our thought processes, our powers of observation and awareness, our focus on the job in hand, our choices and our decision-making. Practices that work with focus, awareness and meditation are all exercising our Light Chakras.

All yoga practices help to harmonize the energies of the Chakras and to maximize their combined energies.

Life energies The three Chakras in the abdominal cavity are concerned with vitality or Life energies. These include the energies that operate in the reproductive system to prepare for, conceive and create a baby, and the energies in the digestive system that nourish the body (and fetus) and clear away the waste products. These systems all lie in the abdominal cavity. Quite a lot of our prenatal yoga practice is aimed at enhancing vitality, to facilitate conception and later to make more space in the abdominal area as the baby grows larger. We also focus on the spinal and pelvic muscles that hold the reproductive organs in place and on bringing vitality to the whole reproductive system.

◁ Spinal stretching for alignment is always an important part of yoga practice as it encourages the flow of energy through the Chakras. This aspect needs special attention during pregnancy as the body shape and weight are constantly changing.

opening your body for pregnancy

Whether you are trying to conceive or are already pregnant, it is vital to remain open at all levels. A woman is probably at her most welcoming at this time, offering her love, her body, her womb, her breasts, her nurturing ability, her home and her whole self as a safe haven. This openness is the pinnacle of femininity – and no experience could be more feminine than welcoming and nurturing the baby growing in your womb. Yoga for conception and pregnancy focuses on staying open and creating more space – more space in the lower abdomen for the baby, more space for the digestive organs to process the food needed by mother and baby, more space for the lungs to provide oxygen for mother and baby.

letting energy flow freely

Openness is a yielding, welcoming quality, but it is not a shapeless "giving in", nor a collapse, for it is literally backed-up by the strength and support of the spine. A key focus in yoga for both conception and pregnancy is to increase and maintain the alignment of the spinal and pelvic bones in order to provide free flow of vital energies and to protect the growing baby. This is vital for several reasons:

• To enable all the systems of the body to perform their functions without pressure or congestion. This is especially important when you are planning to conceive.

"Open the window in the centre of your chest and let spirit move in and out."

Rumi

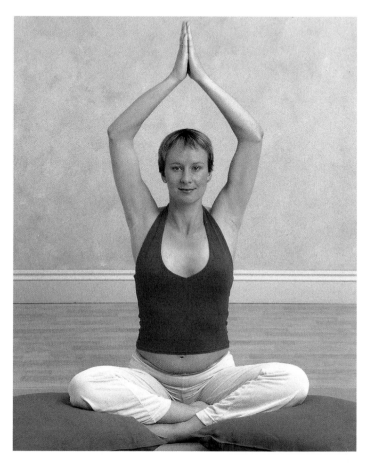

△ In many poses, cushions placed under the knees protect your ligaments from undue strain.

• To hold the baby in place, to create space for movement as he or she develops, and to make room for vital nourishment to pass through the placenta to the baby without any hindrance.

• To allow free passage through the spine of energies that activate the Chakras, as well as the mechanisms that are vital for the smooth running of the nervous system.

All our bones are held in place by muscles and ligaments. Muscles need to be exercised in order to remain strong and flexible and to have the stamina to go on doing their job for as long as necessary. Muscles that are not exercised at first become stiff and then atrophy, which can lead to greater fat deposits. The muscles that support our body's weight are the biggest and strongest ones. In classical yoga, we exercise them a great deal by doing standing poses where the weight of the trunk is taken by gravity through the legs and feet, which are firmly planted on the floor. In pregnancy, however, movement and rhythm are introduced to avoid the strain of holding

THE THREE MAIN STAGES OF PREGNANCY

Here you can see how the spine changes shape and the organs get increasingly squashed. Yoga helps to keep the organs working well and strengthens the all-important, supportive spine.

At 8 weeks

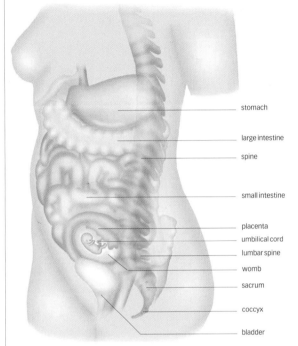

stomach

large intestine

spine

small intestine

placenta
umbilical cord
lumbar spine

womb

sacrum

coccyx

bladder

At 24 weeks

At 40 weeks

the classical positions. Various supports may also be used, to avoid tiring or straining while standing. Many poses are performed either sitting down (less tiring than standing) or lying down (where gravity works with you and the ground supports you).

posture and breathing

Yoga creates a virtuous circle whereby the more you become aware of good posture and alignment of the spine, the more you will pull yourself up whenever you notice you are drooping. The more you stand tall, the better you will breathe and the more vitality you will have. The more vitality you have, the less you will droop and the more you will naturally stand well and move with a spring in your step. Yoga is a holistic discipline, so improvement in any area affects all other areas for the better.

◁ Poor posture can spark all kinds of problems. Compression of the spine leads to pain in the neck and upper back as well as the lower back, while poor breathing from congestion of the lung space inevitably contributes to tiredness and low vitality. Slack abdominal and pelvic muscles lead to congestion in the abdomen and possibly lower back pain and swollen ankles.

▷ Good posture means that your head and neck are erect and balanced between the shoulders, and your spine and pelvis are properly aligned. Your abdominal and pelvic muscles are strong enough to support the baby and your chest is open so that the breathing muscles perform fully and fill the body with a positive vitality. Finally, your legs are strong, springy and balanced.

Yoga after giving birth

Your aim is to use the core aspects of yoga to bring you to a state of full health and vigour, starting from where you are now, soon after giving birth. You can expect to:
• Regain strength in the pelvic and abdominal regions.
• Relax and enjoy deep rest, to compensate for lack of sleep.
• Tone the body back into perfect alignment of hips and spine.
• Learn and practise self-nurture, so that you can nurture and enjoy your baby.

"Each birth, each baby, each mother, is unique."

start at the beginning

Right now you may be feeling very well, or you may have all sorts of problems resulting from hormonal imbalances, poor muscle tone or lack of sleep. However you are feeling, please start at the beginning of this book. The stages are carefully worked out to take you safely from your present postnatal state to your personal maximum level of well-being. Many of the problems that women face in later life – such as uterine prolapse or incontinence – can be traced back to lack of care after childbirth. They are usually avoidable, through an awareness of posture and the right kind of progressive exercise after childbirth. Don't worry about your figure at this stage. It will be regained, perhaps improved, by inside toning.

posture

Regaining good posture is especially important after the birth. The abdominal muscles become very stretched during pregnancy. They may have been cut. Until they are healed and strengthened they cannot hold the spine firmly in place. New mothers need to take special care of the lower back.

△ Standing in Tadasana (28), tilt your pelvis forward and backward slightly. Feel the link between your pelvic floor muscles and both your abdominal and lower back muscles.

◁ Use a futon or a firm bed, with cushions for extra support, for breathing and relaxation practice. It is comfortable for your baby, too.

▷ As your baby grows and you regain strength, it is best to use an upright chair for breathing practice. Always make sure that your knees are level with your hips, using support to raise your feet if needed.

This book teaches you how to move with greater awareness, and to use your legs and upper back to sit and stand, to lift and carry. You then progress safely into gentle movements which build up into flowing sequences to gradually strengthen the weakened and overstretched muscles. Too much vigorous exercise, too soon, would simply strain them further. Full classical yoga postures should not be taken up until the after-effects of the pregnancy and birth have disappeared. It usually takes about six months to reach this stage.

what you need for yoga

Your body needs support, so that you are relaxed and comfortable as you practise. Keep a supply of cushions next to you. For breathing and relaxation you can use your bed, a futon, a firm armchair, or a long sofa. For movement and postures you will need a non-slip mat, measuring about 1 x 2m/3 x 6ft, that you keep just for your yoga practice. If you don't wish to buy one specially, you can use any suitable rug or piece of carpet.

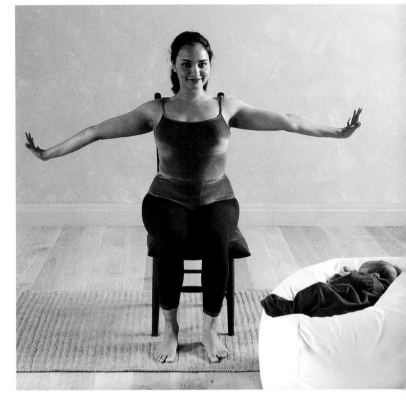

Ideally, it is best to create a special "yoga space" in your home. This trains your mind in the yoga habit and helps you to maintain regular discipline. The good vibrations put you into the right frame of mind as soon as you enter this space, which makes it easy and enjoyable to settle down to regular practice and enjoy your progress.

You can practise relaxation after a heavy meal, but everything else is best done before a meal if possible, or after a light snack. Always wear loose clothes that do not constrict the abdomen, and take off your shoes and socks, so that energy can flow freely around your body.

You do not always have to find the time to install yourself in your "yoga space" or on a special mat or chair to practice yoga. If you cannot manage a practise that day, then just a few minutes of yoga can help you. No effort, no matter how small, is wasted in yoga. The aim of this book is to help you to integrate yoga into your daily life as a new mother, both in your home and outside it.

◁ A futon gives firm support for relaxation, and a beanbag and an upright chair will also be useful. Keep a special mat for your yoga practice. A belt can help your stretches.

healthy
conception

Conception is a miracle of energy, timing and receptivity. These qualities are enhanced through regular yoga practice, which improves the smooth functioning of the reproductive system. Then, when a ripe ovum (egg) is claimed by an eager sperm and slips into the prepared, waiting womb, the two will fuse into one and a unique new person can grow within the nurturing embrace of the mother's body.

How yoga can help you conceive

Stress can impede conception because it ties up so much of our vital energy – and this is detrimental. If stress is claiming energy for keeping our muscles uptight, our minds on overload and our emotions all churned up, the other systems of the body have to manage on the energy that is left over. If conception is eluding you, stress is the most likely culprit. Indeed, long-term stress can even cause medical problems that require medical solutions. Regular yoga practice is a simple preventative measure and can also be a cure. It increases your energy supply and channels it to all the body's systems to keep them in balance so that you become fit and relaxed, living each moment to the full.

what your body language tells you

The way you sit, stand and move can reveal a lot about your state of mind, health and emotional well-being at any time. If most of your energy is tied up either in your mind (your work, for example), in your emotions (say, problems that may be weighing on your mind) or in your hectic lifestyle, your body becomes depleted. There just may not be enough energy left over to work your reproductive system properly. It can be as simple as that. This stress can be reflected in your body language – legs tightly crossed, upper spine hunched over, or arms crossed over your chest.

"This state, in which the senses are steady and at rest, is known as yoga, the state of union."

Katha Upanishad VI 9

The yogic answer to stress is to rebalance your nervous and endocrine systems so that all functions are enhanced. Use yoga to stretch, strengthen, open and relax. This releases locked-up energy, and so eases conception, pregnancy and birth.

△ The "uptight" body language here says it all. This posture displays feelings of fear and vulnerability. The arms and legs form a shield across the trunk, blocking the flow of energy. The chest and abdomen are closed, so that breathing is restricted and energy to the pelvic area is blocked.

△ The body language here shows a relaxed mind, peaceful emotions and an erect, vibrant spine. The shoulders, neck, hips and pelvis are relaxed so that energy can flow freely throughout the body.

breath is the key

The respiratory and cardiovascular systems bring oxygen (the prime source of energy) into the body from the outside air and circulate it to every cell. Good breathing habits, therefore, increase the total supply of energy available for the body's systems to use. The diaphragm is the large muscle that separates the abdomen from the chest cavity. It is the chief breathing muscle. If its movement is restricted through poor posture it cannot pump enough air into the lungs and so not enough oxygen is available to the body. Shallow breathing, which does not draw in enough oxygen, is one of the main causes of feeling below par. Deep breathing (using the diaphragm fully) is instantly energizing.

As you breathe in, the diaphragm contracts strongly downwards, massaging and energizing the abdominal organs and increasing lung capacity so that air rushes in, through the nose, from outside. The diaphragm springs back up again as you breathe out, releasing the abdominal pressure and decreasing the lung capacity so that air is forced out through the nose. This contraction and release reflects the whole momentum of yoga – activity followed by rest, followed by activity, in a continuous, balanced cycle. Practised with awareness, deep breathing reconnects us with this rhythm of life and helps us to learn how to relax deeply between all bouts of activity. It also helps to create a calm strength.

1 Tuning in to your breath

A deep breath in recharges both body and mind. A deep breath out releases muscular tension, chemical waste products and tired, strained feelings. Mentally, take your breath in to the very base of your spine. Taking time to practise breathing slowly, deeply and fully induces calm, positive feelings.

◁ Sit at the back of a firm chair with spine erect, knees apart and feet on the floor. Rest your hands with palms up in an open, receptive gesture. This position opens the trunk, so the diaphragm can move freely. Take several deep breaths with awareness of what is happening to your body as you breathe. Repeat the exercise frequently.

CAUTION
Deep breathing is strenuous, especially if it is new to you. Stop at once if you feel tired, breathless or light-headed. Rest for a while before starting again. Very gradually build up the number of deep breaths you take at any one time.

2 Flexibility in the pelvis

The reproductive system lies within the lower part of the abdomen and is protected by the bony pelvic girdle. This area needs to be open and relaxed so that energy can circulate freely through the reproductive system and conception is unhindered. Regular movement of the pelvis brings energy, flexibility and strength to this area.

◁ **1** Sit on the edge of a sturdy chair with feet apart and set firmly on the floor. Place your hands on your thighs above your knees, with fingers turned in and elbows turned out. Lean forward, bend your elbows and take your upper body weight on your thighs. This frees the pelvis – think of it as a bowl and tip it forward at the front "rim" (the pubic bone) and up at the back "rim" (where the sacrum joins the spine).

▷**2** Open the front of the body by spreading your arms with palms up, lifting your chest and tucking your pelvis under so that the front pelvic "rim" rises and the back "rim" is lowered. This movement stretches the spine and releases tension. It also tightens the lower abdominal muscles that hold the pelvis in place. Repeat these two movements several times and practise frequently in order to increase mobility in the

healthy conception

breath awareness

As well as energizing the body, our breathing has a profound influence on the nervous system. Fast or shallow breathing makes us feel anxious and stressed, whereas slow, deep breathing immediately relaxes us. If you are to practise active relaxation, you need to be aware of your breathing patterns, so that you can use your breath to consciously reduce stress and promote well-being. Note that the awareness of exhalation comes first in yoga, avoiding any forceful inhalation.

3 Deepening the breath

Sit upright on a sturdy chair, with your feet apart and planted firmly on the floor. Feel your breathing muscles working by placing your hands on your ribs, then lower chest, then abdomen. The lower you can take the breathing movement the more energized and relaxed you will feel, and the more efficiently your abdominal organs (digestive and reproductive) can function. In yoga you should always breathe in and out through the nose unless instructed otherwise.

△ **1** Bring your elbows back to open your chest, and place your hands on the sides of your ribs with fingers pointing forward. Breathe in deeply, expanding your ribcage against your hands. Breathe out, keeping the lift and openness in the chest. Be careful not to collapse, even though your ribcage contracts a little. Repeat several times.

△ **2** Still with elbows wide and chest open, bring your hands forward with fingers pointing towards each other and little fingers against your lowest ribs. As you breathe in feel your lower ribs expanding outwards and your diaphragm contracting downwards against your abdominal organs. As you breathe out feel the ribs relaxing inwards and the diaphragm relaxing upwards. Repeat several times. Blow the air out forcibly through your mouth and feel the corset muscles around your waist contracting sharply.

△ **3** Move your hands below the navel to feel the effect of deep breathing on the abdominal organs. As you breathe in, contracting the diaphragm, the downward pressure massages and flushes away stale blood from these organs. As you breathe out this pressure is released and fresh blood rushes in, bringing a new supply of oxygen and nutrients. Feel the movements reaching right down through the abdomen to the muscular pelvic floor. Repeat a few times, keeping neck and shoulders relaxed, and then rest.

4 Stretch, bend and relax

This exercise sets the pattern for all your yoga practice – alternating active movements with a pause to relax. If you can arrange your daily life to the same natural rhythm you will find that you can undo stress before it has a chance to build up. Either sitting or standing you can rid the lungs of stale air, open the chest and massage the abdominal organs.

△ **1** Make sure you are seated comfortably. Use a firm bolster or similar as a foot support. Breathe in and raise both straight arms above your head.

△ **2** As you breathe out fold forward like a rag doll, dropping your head between your knees and hands loosely to the floor.

△ **3** Breathing naturally, relax your neck and shoulders to ease out any tension. Repeat this exercise several times.

5 Lengthening the outbreath

The breath out relaxes the nervous system, whereas the breath in is energizing. First, sigh or yawn to release tension. Always remember to make the breath out last a little longer than the breath in. An enjoyable way to lengthen the breath out is by using the voice. A lower pitch usually resonates better than a higher one and is more relaxing.

▷ With spine erect and chest open, breathe in deeply and let the air out slowly as you chant "A...E...I...O...U...".

6 Alternate nostril breathing

This breathing exercise is a classical yoga practice. It is remarkable for soothing the nervous system and balancing our extrovert and introvert tendencies – calming us when we are anxious or overexcited and lifting our spirits when we are tired or depressed. Ideally, it should be practised for a few minutes each day.

▷ Sit with spine erect and chest open. Place the right hand in front of the face, with the index and middle finger resting lightly on the centre of the forehead, the thumb in position to close the right nostril, and the ring finger in position to close the left nostril. Now concentrate and follow these steps:

- Close the right nostril with the thumb and breathe in through the left.
- Close the left nostril and open the right.
- Breathe out through the right nostril.
- Breathe in through the right nostril.
- Close the right nostril and open the left.
- Breathe out through the left nostril.

Repeat, gradually building up the number of rounds over a few weeks.

Yoga poses to *release* tension

For many people, tension seems to settle in the pelvic region, causing stiffness in the hips, pain in the lower back, and general congestion and an uptight feeling in the lower abdominal area. Yoga stretches relieve all these conditions and allow energy to circulate freely once more. They also work on the whole body, so remember to keep the spine extended and the chest open in all these exercises.

CAUTION
Make haste slowly. Widen your legs and stretch to the side and forwards only as far as you comfortably can. Locked-in tension impedes movement and should never be fought against. As you release the tension through yoga movements, you will find it easier to move much further and to relax more deeply into the positions. All yoga stretching should be performed with active relaxation and not force or effort.

7 Seated looseners

Let your partner encourage and help you. It is fun and relaxing for both of you. The closeness of trying to conceive can permeate all aspects of your life together.

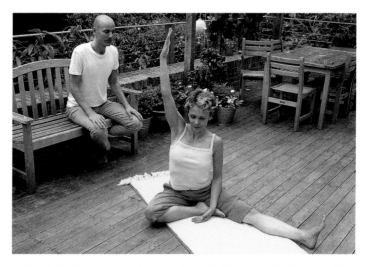

△ **1** Sit on the floor (on a yoga mat or piece of non-slip carpet) with legs extended and feet comfortably far apart. Bend your right knee and bring your foot to rest against your left inner thigh, with your heel as close to the pubic bone as possible. Flex your left ankle and straighten your left knee. Raise your right arm overhead and stretch up through your right side, breathing in.

△ **2** Breathe out as you lean to the left over your left leg, with your left arm sliding gently along your leg and your right arm stretching up. Breathe in as you sit up, lowering your right arm.

△ **3** Breathe out as you bend to the right, walking your hands along the floor each side of your bent right leg. Keep the left ankle flexed and stretch right through your left side as you bend over your right leg. Breathe in as you sit up straight. Repeat a few times on the same side. Then breathe naturally as you

8 Kneeling looseners

Loosening movements can also be performed using a sofa or bench for leverage, so that you can get a strong twist in the upper body while keeping your spine extended and erect, and hips in position.

△ **1** Kneel with your right side against the bench, then raise your right leg and place it along the bench seat. Flex your ankle. Hold the back of the bench and breathe in. Breathe out, pulling your upper body around to the right, with your spine erect and chest open. Breathe in and face forward.

△ **2** Place your right hand against your inner right leg and use the arm of the bench to lever your upper body round to the left as you breathe out. Breathe in to face forward again.

△ **3** Breathe out to lean forward and slide your upturned hands alongside your straight right leg. Breathe in as you sit up straight. Repeat these movements a few times on the same side, then turn around and repeat to stretch the other side.

9 Happy womb poses

It is important to focus your attention in the lower abdomen and to create space there in order to bring more energy to the reproductive system. Sit on the floor or a chair and open your hips, with your knees wide apart, as often as possible. You can sit comfortably on the floor to read, talk on the phone, watch TV and do most of those things you normally do sitting in a chair – only in a chair the pelvic area is apt to be constricted, especially if you cross your legs.

◁ **1** Lie on your back, bend your knees and hold a knee in each hand. Keeping your chin tucked down and your waist against the floor (using the abdominal muscles). Rotate your knees outwards with your hands, relaxing and opening the hip joints. Circle the knees out and in again several times.

△ **2** Sit upright, legs loosely crossed and a scarf around your middle, crossed over at the abdomen. As you breathe out pull the scarf ends gently to create pressure. Breathe in deeply against this pressure to open the scarf and bring the breathing movements down into the lower abdomen and pelvic floor. Repeat several times.

△ **3** Sit with your knees bent and your feet apart and flat on the floor. Now bring your palms together with bent elbows. Keeping your chest open, gently press your elbows against your inner thighs for a few moments to open the hip joints. Breathe slowly and deeply.

△ **4** Remaining seated, lean forward and place your hands on the floor with palms upwards. Gently press your knees apart with your upper arms. Breathe deeply, lengthening the out-breath for as long as you can.

Nearly effortless stretches

healthy conception

Physical movement increases blood flow, and therefore the supply of oxygen, to the part of the body that is being moved – bringing new fuel (and thus energy) to the cellular structures. This blood flow also removes accumulated waste products, which can cause harmful imbalances if allowed to build up.

Awareness focused on any part of the body also brings vital energy to that part, since energy follows thought. The following exercises are done lying down because this allows maximum relaxation of the nervous system.

10 Pelvic movements with focused awareness

These relaxing movements encourage increased awareness, blood flow and flexibility in the pelvic area. Feel that you are opening up to new healing energy and letting go of any tension there.

◁ **1** Lie on your back, with a large book and three cushions. Place one cushion under your head and tuck your chin in to lengthen the back of your neck. Bend your knees and plant your feet hip-width apart on the floor. Place the book on your lower abdomen, evenly balanced on the hip bones and the pubic bone, then stretch your arms alongside your body with the palms down to support you.

△ **2** As you breathe in press on your hands and arch your lower back as much as you can, so that the navel and hip bones rise and the front "rim" of your pelvis (and the book) is tipped towards your feet.

△ **3** As you breathe out pull the navel against the spine and press on your hands to lift the coccyx just off the floor, so that the pelvic front "rim" (and the book) is now tipped backward, towards your head. Keep your waist against the floor and move the lower spine only. Repeat steps 1–3 several times.

△ **4** Now place your hands, in a relaxed pose, on top of the book and breathe deeply. Feel the movements of the book over the pelvic area as you breathe in and out slowly for several minutes.

△ **5** Remove the book and bring the soles of your feet together so that your knees fall outward. Support them with the remaining two cushions. Place your hands, palms up, beside you in a gesture of openness and complete surrender. Relax for several minutes.

11 Improving flexibility and muscle tone

Here are three simple exercises to improve flexibility in the spine and hips and to strengthen the abdominal muscles. They may seem strenuous to begin with, but strength and flexibility will improve rapidly with practice. Relax afterwards and feel the effects of the exercises on your muscles and your breath. Keep your coccyx on the floor throughout.

▷ **1** Lie on your back with a cushion under your head and your arms, palms down, alongside the body to support you. Bend your right leg, keeping your left leg stretched with the ankle flexed. Make large cycling circles with your right leg until you feel tired. Then rest with both legs stretched out and become aware of the muscles you have been working in the right side of the lower abdomen. Repeat the same number of circles with your left leg, and then rest again.

△ **2** With your left knee bent and left foot planted firmly on the floor, take hold of your right knee and move the right leg in circles from the hip. This releases tightness in the groin and hip joint. Rest, then repeat on the other side.

△ **3** Now work with both knees and the breath. Breathe in as you take the knees out to the sides. Breathe out as you pull your knees close to your chest to stretch your lower back. Repeat several times then rest.

12 Lying twist

This powerful but simple twisting exercise opens up and relaxes both the shoulders and the hips. This in turn helps to make the entire spine more flexible, creating space between the vertebrae.

▷ Lie down, raise your arms, bent at the elbows, and place them on the floor above or beside your head. This position opens and lifts the chest. Bend your knees and place your feet together on the floor. Breathe in. As you breathe out lower both knees to the right, ensuring that you keep them together. The aim is to place your right knee on the floor without letting your left elbow leave the floor, but only take it as far as feels comfortable. As you breathe in raise your knees to the centre, still keeping them pressed together. As you breathe out lower them to the left and raise them again as you breathe in. Repeat until tired, then relax for several minutes.

Sharing energy with your partner

Do you lack quality time with your partner? It may be that you are both so busy that you hardly ever have time simply to enjoy each other's company. Yogic stretching, relaxing and unwinding together may be all that is needed to make your womb, and his sperm, more "conception friendly".

Nature often works on a subliminal level and an openness and emotional intimacy with each other can increase the likelihood of conception. Remember too, that prolonged stress can adversely affect the reproductive systems of both sexes, and that

yoga gradually dissolves the effects of past stress and also helps to prevent new stress from building up.

Couples are very often disappointed if conception does not occur exactly when they are ready for it, especially as preparing for a baby involves great shifts in outlook and investments of energy. Yoga helps to deepen harmony and acceptance between hopeful parents at this difficult stage.

▷ **Teach your partner the joys of yoga relaxation. Stress affects his reproductive capabilities too.**

13 Moving energy into your reproductive system

Every single message passing along your nervous system between the brain and the body has to go through the neck. It is hardly surprising that the neck and shoulders often get tense and energy-congested. Massage releases this congestion and allows energy to move freely around the body once again.

△ Ask your partner to massage your neck and shoulders to restore energy flow while you place your hands on your abdomen and focus on "charging" your ovaries with deep breathing.

14 Synchronizing your energies

When both partners are relaxed, synchronized and emotionally ready for conception – "two hearts beating as one" – a favourable energy field will help conception to take place.

◁ **1** Sit back to back so that the flow of energy in your spines can synchronize, bringing you closer together on an energy level. You will find that your breathing also synchronizes as you relax into each other and become much more intimate.

◁ **2** To become even closer, sit facing each other with spines straight. Place your legs over your partner's legs, snuggle up, place your palms against his and gaze into each other's eyes. Your energies will synchronize and pass from one to the other through your eyes and your joined palms.

A sample practice for promoting conception

1

▷ Tuning in to your breath (1)

2 △ Happy womb pose (9)

3

◁ Deepening the breath (3)

4

◁ Stretch, bend and relax (4)

6

▷ Lengthening the outbreath (5)

5 △ Pelvic movements with focused awareness (10)

Questions and answers

• **Roughly how long should we try to conceive before consulting medical experts?**

If you have been taking oral contraceptives for years and then stop in order to conceive, your reproductive system may take up to a year to re-establish its natural rhythm. If you and your partner have stressful jobs you may need to take steps to change your lifestyles so that you can both reduce your stress levels. Yoga practice speeds up the rate at which you de-stress. Medical intervention may ultimately be needed but remember that medical procedures are in themselves stressful – so do what you can to help yourselves first. Remember also that there is no definite answer – everyone is different.

• **We have had all the medical tests recommended to us and there is nothing wrong with either of us. What can we do now?**

If both of you have undergone tests that have revealed nothing, there may be simple reasons why you have not conceived yet. The most common reason is simply that it can take a long time – always far too long when you are waiting eagerly. Highly subtle psychological and physiological changes can make a difference here. For example, the slight shifts in pH levels – in both you and your partner – that can arise from continued yoga and relaxation practices, could help to lead you further down the road to conception.

• **What are the chances of success with IVF procedures?**

Only medical experts can advise you in your particular case. IVF procedures are increasingly successful.

• **I just can't relax. What am I doing wrong?**

Getting uptight about relaxing in order to conceive! It is better to learn to relax in order to reduce the stress in your life. This then creates an atmosphere where conception becomes more likely. Go on holiday with your partner and practise yoga together away from your daily routine. Make plans to simplify your lives when you get home so that you can enjoy more quality time together. Make yoga part of your life and use your positive affirmations each day. Most importantly, affirm your blessings with regard to what you already have in life.

• **I have a specific medical problem (such as having just one ovary) that makes conception difficult.**

A positive attitude is a great help in overcoming all kinds of obstacles, but we also have to cultivate an open, accepting disposition that will enable us to embrace our life equally well if conception remains elusive. Seek expert medical help and keep as healthy and relaxed as possible. Use regular yogic exercise, breathing, relaxation and meditation practices to keep all the systems of your body running as smoothly as possible.

1–14
weeks

Congratulations on becoming
pregnant! Right from the moment
of conception, Nature's first priority
is the welfare of the fetus growing in
the womb. Your own needs take
second place now. While your body is
adjusting to this totally new situation –
which can take up to 14 weeks – your
hormonal balance is fragile, so it is
important to conserve your energy and
to respond to your body's needs rather
than trying to ignore them.

Make space in your life for your pregnancy

No doubt you already realize that you will have to re-arrange your priorities once your baby is born. However, the best time to start is right now. Making a baby requires a lot of energy, but our energy is limited, especially if we lead busy lives. That energy must come from somewhere and therefore, since Nature ensures that your baby comes first and gets all it needs to develop, it is vital that you conserve and boost your own energy levels. Yoga conserves energy by reducing stress through deep relaxation and boosts it by increasing your oxygen uptake through yogic deep breathing and movement.

get the yoga habit now

Yoga will stand you in good stead right through your pregnancy, after your baby is born and for the rest of your life. You will soon be hooked on the sense of well-being that it brings. Your daily session can be quite short, as long as it is regular, and many yoga techniques can be incorporated into daily life. As you become more aware of your posture, emotions, thoughts and attitudes, you will want to adjust them, whatever you happen to be doing and wherever you are.

learn to nurture yourself

Many women feel that they should hide their feelings, ignore their needs, always appear strong and independent and keep going, no matter what. But you must learn to stop, relax and nurture yourself. Only when you know what it feels like to be loved will you have the capacity to nurture the life in your womb and care for a tiny baby. Practise being vulnerable and learn to ask for help and support from your loved ones.

CAUTION
Whether or not you have practised yoga before, keep it very easy and simple for the first 14 weeks of your pregnancy. Focus on breathing and relaxation rather than movement.

15 Feet up the wall sequence

This relaxing sequence rests tired legs and lower back, while stretching the muscles in the groin and preparing the muscles of the pelvic floor. Meanwhile, practise slow, deep breathing with awareness.

△1 Sit with the legs along a wall. Bend the inner knee, lean back on the hands and then forearms, and swivel round before raising the legs.

△ 2 Swivel your body round and straighten your legs against the wall – buttocks and legs should touch the wall. Put a cushion under your head.

△ 3 Place your hands under your head with elbows on the floor, to open up your chest. Breathe deeply for a few moments.

△ 4 Take your legs comfortably apart to release tightness in the pelvis and groin. Gently massage the inner thighs while breathing deeply.

◁ 5 Bend your knees and slide the soles of your feet down the wall, a comfortable width apart. Place your hands over your lower abdomen and become aware of your pelvic floor muscles. Draw in the muscles as you breathe in, and release the tension gently as you breathe out. Repeat several times.

16 Lying down stretches

A similar exercise helps to relax the pelvic region for conception but it is just as effective here, where the point of focus is the lower back. The lumbar region of the spine, the sacrum and the coccyx should all relax against the floor – quite easy when the knees are bent and pulled gently toward the chest. If muscular tension prevents the lower spine from softening in this position, take long deep breaths out to relax more fully. The gentle movements will further ease your lower back and remove any stiffness or soreness.

△ **1** Lie on your back with your spine long and chin down. Keeping your coccyx on the floor, take one bent knee in each hand. Bring your knees toward your chest then gently circle them out to the sides to massage your lower back against the floor to release backache. Repeat several times.

△ **2** Gently bring one knee toward the floor. As far as possible, make sure that both shoulders remain relaxed and your back stays flat against the floor. Keep your neck relaxed and breathe deeply.

△ **3** Breathe out as you roll on to one side, bringing your knees together. Relax in this position and breathe deeply. Breathe in to roll on to your back, raising first one knee and then the other, or both together if you can. Repeat on the other side.

17 The bridge pose

This pose strengthens the leg muscles, especially the inner thighs, which helps you to support the extra weight of your baby as the pregnancy progresses. The Bridge Pose also stretches the muscles around the groin area, opens the chest and frees the diaphragm for deeper breathing. Alternate this exercise with the previous one so that you both relax and strengthen the lower spine and abdominal muscles. This will bring awareness and energy to the whole area.

△ Place your feet flat on the floor near your buttocks, about hip-width apart. Stretch your arms alongside your body, palms down, for support. Breathe in and raise your pelvis off the floor. Breathe deeply a few times in this position. Slowly lower your buttocks to the floor on a long breath out. Repeat several times.

18 Deep relaxation with focused breathing

Leave enough time so that you can end every yoga session with deep relaxation. It quickly dissolves any stress that may have built up, removing muscular tension and congestion and bringing new energy to all the body's systems.

◁ **2** Place your palms over your lower abdomen, thumbs touching. Breathe deeply, and feel which is the best hand position to soothe you and bring nourishment to your baby. Close your eyes and relax.

△ **1** Lie on your back with your spine long and chin down. Drape your legs over a beanbag or a pile of cushions, with knees bent out to the sides. Bring your heels close together and relax your feet.

A strong, supple spine supports your baby

Good posture is especially important during pregnancy for the following reasons.

• It holds your womb, in which your baby lies, in its correct position in the lower abdomen. This makes your pregnancy a far more comfortable experience for both of you.

• It relieves backache and can avoid its onset.

• It creates more space in the chest and abdominal areas, which become increasingly crowded by the presence of the growing baby.

• It improves breathing, and therefore your energy levels, because it gives the diaphragm more room to move.

• It improves digestion, which cannot function properly if there is compression in the abdomen.

• It prevents congestion in the circulatory system to the womb, upon which your baby depends for all its nourishment.

• It streamlines your figure, however large or small the bump.

• It makes you feel great. Standing and walking tall express a positive outlook, whereas the general compression and congestion that result from poor posture can make your energy stagnate and your mood depressed.

Although changes to your figure may be hard to detect in the early days, especially in your first pregnancy, it is important to concentrate on your posture from the start, before any bad habits are established.

19 Dog pose

This pose lengthens the spine and increases spinal awareness, as well as strengthening the muscles in the upper back, arms and hands. It also improves circulation and releases tension across the shoulders, and in the neck and face. Below are three variations on the Dog Pose. Try them all out and see which one suits you best.

▷ **Pose 1** Hold on to a table, stool or radiator and step away from it until your spine and arms are stretched and horizontal to the floor, and your feet are hip-width apart. It helps initially if someone checks that your back is flat. Keep your head and neck horizontal, so that your ears are in line with your arms. Breathe deeply and bend your knees slightly if this helps you stretch further.

△ **Pose 2** Make a right angle by walking your hands forward (shoulder-width apart) with knees bent. Straighten your legs (feet hip-width apart) on a breath out, bringing your heels to the floor if you can. As you breathe in stretch through the spine and arms. Hold the pose for a few breaths, breathing deeply.

△ **Pose 3** From the position shown in Pose 2, balance on one leg and raise the other. Keep the knee of the leg that is on the floor bent. Push down into your arms and hands. Now change legs to repeat on the other side.

20 Alignment of the spine

Your posture can be improved simply by becoming aware and straightening up whenever you notice that you are drooping. The back of the body, being bonier than the front, has less sensation (fewer nerve endings), so it is quite difficult to be aware of the position of your spine. It helps to stand or sit against a surface such as a wall, so you can feel whether your muscles are holding your spine firmly upright or are slack. With practice, both awareness and posture will improve as you locate and strengthen the relevant muscles.

△ **1** Stand with feet a short distance from the wall and hands behind your waist. Press against the wall. Lengthen your neck, lowering your chin. Breathe in and stand as tall as you can. Hold this stretch and contact with the wall as you breathe out. Repeat a few times.

△ **2** Now bring your heels and calves against the wall and repeat the same stretch up as you breathe in, maintaining contact with the wall as you breathe out. Repeat.

△ **3** Bring your hands to your sides and press your waist against the wall as you stretch up, breathing in. Maintain contact with the wall as you breathe out. Repeat.

△ **4** Bend one knee and clasp both hands around your shin. Draw your thigh close to your chest as you breathe out, balancing the other leg. Release the pull on your shin as you breathe in and stretch up, keeping contact with the wall. Repeat.

△ **5** Sit on a low stool with knees apart and feet firmly planted on the floor. Maintain contact with the wall with your head, shoulders, waist and buttocks as you breathe in and stretch up, then breathe out and hold the upward stretch.

△ **6** Once you have found and strengthened your spinal muscles, practise lifting up through your spine whenever you are standing or sitting.

Easy standing poses

1–14 weeks

Now that you have learnt how to keep your spine aligned, and know how good that feels, you can maintain the alignment as you move gracefully through these sequences. They develop strength and suppleness, helping you to protect and nourish your growing baby as well as yourself. They also help to keep your feet firmly on the ground and remain steady as your body changes.

21 Grounding

The joints and muscles around your hips, legs and feet take the weight of your whole body, and the muscles of the pelvis and pelvic floor carry the weight of your upper body and trunk. These important muscle groups can be strengthened and toned by the following grounding exercise, which allows your weight to pass smoothly through your legs and feet into the ground beneath you. It becomes ever more important to work with gravity rather than against it as your baby becomes heavier.

△ **1** Stand with your feet apart and loosely bend your knees, making sure you maintain your upright posture through the spine.

△ **2** Bring your hands into Namaste, the prayer position, and press your palms firmly together with elbows out to the sides.

△ **3** Spread your hands wide, so that you keep your elbows bent and open up your chest area, all the time breathing in deeply.

◁ **4** Stretch your arms out to the sides and lower them, breathing out. Repeat steps 1 to 4 several times.

▷ **5** For a stronger version of this exercise, place one foot on a low chair and bend the other knee. Change legs after a few breaths and repeat with the other foot on the chair.

22 Standing stretches

By stretching up from the hips and through the waist, these stretches create space for the diaphragm to contract downwards to a greater extent, so that you breathe more deeply. Twist and sway rhythmically as if you are dancing.

◁ **1** Stand with knees loosely bent and stretch your arms overhead, first one side and then the other. Feel your ribs and waist opening and releasing.

▷ **2** Now bring your arms out at shoulder level and swing round from the waist, first to one side and then the other, without changing your leg or arm position. Repeat both movements.

23 Adapted easy triangle sequence

This sequence works out your oblique abdominal muscles and your lumbar spine. Strong obliques help to prevent backache, hold your developing baby firmly and trim your figure.

△ **1** Stand tall with feet wide and knees bent. Place your hands on your hips and sway from side to side, tipping your pelvis up to the right as you sway to the right and up to the left as you sway to the left in a rhythmical movement. Keep spine erect, coccyx tucked under and chest lifted. Repeat several times to loosen the hips and pelvis.

△ **2** Bend to your right side without tipping forward. Place your right hand along your leg and bring your left elbow back to open the left side of the waist and chest as you look upwards.

△ **3** Now stretch your left arm right up and back to open the left side of your body. Repeat the movement while bending to your left side. Repeat several times on each side.

Greater challenges

An erect spine, an open chest and awareness of the position of your body and the flow of your energy are the fundamentals of yoga practice. Standing and sitting tall, at all times, will quickly improve your grace and posture and also help to prevent backache and digestive problems, while daily practice of deep breathing with awareness will soon make this your natural way to breathe. These simple practices are also the basis from which you can go on to develop more challenging yoga poses.

24 Adapted easy tree pose

This is a balancing pose requiring good posture, steady deep breathing, stillness and focus. Start with the simpler versions of this pose and work up to the classical pose in your own time. All balancing poses create inner calm and poise as well as physical stillness. Standing tall and balanced becomes more difficult as the baby grows out to the front, so it is important to develop your balancing muscles from the beginning of your pregnancy in order to maintain your grace and poise throughout it.

◁ **1** Stand with a wall on your right side. Stretch both arms to the sides at shoulder level. Rest your right hand against the wall for balance. Stand tall with chest open and coccyx tucked under. Bend your left knee and balance on your right foot. Now place your left sole against the inside of your right leg and bring your left knee to the side, opening up the left hip without compromising your erect posture. The aim is to get your knee out to the left so that you can push your sole high up against the right groin, without tilting your pelvis. Practise on one side then the other.

> **CAUTION**
> Make sure you keep your base foot straight and resist swaying to the side of your standing leg.

△ **2** Place a low stool in front of you. Place your left foot on the stool and bring your palms together in Namaste, the prayer position, in front of your sternum. Stand tall and gaze at a point in front of you, breathing steadily and deeply.

△ **3** Take your left foot off the stool and place the sole against your inner right leg. Use your left hand to help you find a good position for your foot, then return to the Namaste position and breath deeply. Come out of the position smoothly.

△ **4** This is the classical pose. Place your heel against the groin with the knee out to the side. Focus on your breath and then join your palms together high above your head. Take a few good breaths while in this position, and then relax.

25 Pushing hands

It is fun to practise yoga with a friend, so that you can help each other with your posture. Of course, you can also use a wall if you wish.

▷ Stand tall, with arms outstretched and palms together. Each person takes a step forward with one leg (you can use either the same or the opposite leg to your partner). Keeping upright, with your hips facing forward, press your palms against those of your partner. Use comfortable pressure as you press, and, as you do so, breathe as deeply as you can and feel the involvement of your abdominal muscles. Change legs and repeat.

26 Classical "cobbler's pose"

This seated position was traditionally used by cobblers and tailors, who needed to use both their hands and also hold things between their feet, and we can still benefit from it today. Many Western women have tight ligaments in the groin and pelvic area, through frequent sitting in a chair or car. It is important to stretch this whole area for ease in giving birth.

Practise sitting on the floor instead of lounging in an easy chair whenever you can – to watch TV, read or chat, for example – and this open position will soon become familiar and comfortable. Place cushions under your knees to begin with, until the groin ligaments stretch and relax naturally. Sit against a wall, or piece of solid furniture, until you can hold your spine erect without discomfort. Once this position feels easy and natural you can also use it to meditate on your baby or to practise deep breathing.

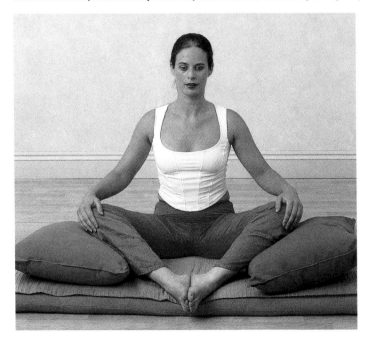

CAUTION
Ligaments need to be stretched gradually and naturally without hurry or forcing. This is especially true during pregnancy, when special hormones gradually soften your ligaments so that they will stretch naturally to allow your baby to be born.

Make yoga a part of your life

There is no special time to practise deep breathing, stretching, relaxation, meditation or quietly observing your body, your feelings and your thoughts. All these are yoga practices that you can do as you go about your daily activities, or fit into those moments when you create a pause between one activity and the next. A few minutes of yogic awareness, frequently repeated, becomes a habit that gradually builds up good health, positive feelings and a clear and focused mind.

27 Sitting position for relaxation and alternate nostril breathing

During the day, you should take a few moments to sit and breathe deeply between one task and the next. Make a conscious decision to change your focus from outer activity to inner silence, so that this becomes a regular rhythm.

Place a comfortable, upright chair, preferably with arms, in a convenient place in your home or office and practise getting into and out of it while keeping your spine stretched and aligned. This may be easy now, but it will become more challenging as your baby grows and the extra weight pulls your lower back into an exaggerated arch, a prime cause of backache. You may need to adjust your sitting position by placing a small cushion between your lumbar arch and the chair, or a stool or cushion under your feet so that they do not hang down without support. If your chair has no arms, place your hands palms up in your lap, or palms down on your thighs.

△ **1** Stand tall in front of your yoga chair, looking ahead with your hands by your side. Your back should be well extended and supportive but relaxed rather than rigid.

△ **2** Now lower yourself carefully on to the chair, keeping your spine extended and using the arms of the chair for support.

△ **3** Sit upright at the back of the chair, with your spine supported. Place your forearms on the chair arms and plant your feet hip-width apart on the floor. Breathe slowly and deeply with eyes closed, moving your focus inward. While in this seated position, practise Alternate Nostril Breathing (6).

28 Stretch the spine with deep breathing

Your kitchen is an excellent place to practise yogic stretches, as it will probably have a work surface that is a useful height, and maybe a high chair or stool. And you can stretch while waiting for the kettle to boil. The whole body benefits from this sequence. Your legs and feet are strengthened in preparation for carrying the extra weight of your growing baby, and the spine is extended to make more room and to allow for deeper breathing and better digestion. The upper back and neck are freed from any build-up of tension and your grace and balance are enhanced.

▷ **1** Place your hands on a work surface and walk away from it, bending at the hips until your trunk is at a right angle to your hips, with as much space as possible between your ribs and your hips. Keep your neck and head level, with your ears between your arms, and your feet a little more than hip-width apart. Breathe slowly and deeply in this position, feeling the diaphragm move.

◁ **2** Breathing out, bend your knees into an easy squat without moving your feet. Come back up on an in breath. Repeat.

▷ **3** If you are able to keep your back straight in a full squat, practise closer to the work surface, breathing fully in the pose.

△ **4** Place a high stool or chair behind you to sit on. Stand tall with your hands on the work surface. Breathe in and take one foot back toward the stool.

△ **5** Raise your arms to shoulder level and breathe out as you lower yourself on to the stool, keeping your spine erect and stretched up.

△ **6** Sit tall on the stool with your hands on your upper thighs and elbows bent to the sides to open your chest and shoulders. Breathe deeply, holding this open position. Stand slowly on an in breath.

relax and meditate with your baby

Focusing upon one thing, so that your heart and mind become peaceful and calm, takes you from deep relaxation into the meditative state. This yogic method is especially fulfilling when you are pregnant, as your baby can become the focus of your meditation. In addition, your baby will benefit enormously from your peaceful state and will relax with you.

This focus on your baby from the very beginning of his or her existence creates a close emotional bond between you even before birth – so that you and your baby are communicating and growing ever closer and more comfortable with each other right from conception. This is especially helpful if you have not had a baby before.

29 Walking meditation

It is important to take a break, with a change of activity and focus, when you have been sitting or doing mental work for a while. Stand up and stretch, then align your spine and go for a gentle walking meditation somewhere quiet, either indoors or outdoors. Your footsteps and breathing will gradually synchronize, taking you deep into yourself and into communion with your baby

◁ Stand tall and walk very slowly, with short, easy steps. Focus on your baby, placing your hands on your lower abdomen, over your womb. As you breathe in, lift your chest and open your heart space to receive the energy this brings. As you breathe out feel that you are giving this energy, and your love, to your baby. After a few moments, bring your attention slowly back to the outside world. Breathe deeply with a sigh or a yawn, stretch your arms overhead, look all around you and focus on the world outside yourself. Then return to daily life, fully refreshed and at peace.

30 Deep relaxation, watching the flow of the breath

It is easiest to relax completely when lying on your back, either with your feet up the wall or with cushions or a beanbag under your knees. If you plan to relax for more than 10 minutes you may want to cover yourself with a blanket or rug, as your body temperature may drop. Get comfortable and settled, close your eyes and breathe deeply and steadily for a few moments. Allow your mind to rest on the sensations of breathing.

◁ Let your attention follow the passage of air in through your nose, deep into your lungs and out again through your nose in a rhythmic, soothing cycle. When you are ready to get up, breathe strongly and deeply before stretching through your whole body and, finally, opening your eyes.

"I am light with meditation…"

Douglas Dunn

A sample practice for the early months

1

▷ Feet up the wall sequence (15)

2

△ Dog pose (19)

3

▷ Grounding (21)

4

◁ Triangle sequence (23)

5

◁ Sitting position for relaxation and alternate nostril breathing (27)

6

△ Deep relaxation with focused breathing (18)

Questions and answers

• **I suffer from severe nausea. Is there anything I can do about this?**
Nausea is a common problem while your hormonal system is adjusting to the requirements of pregnancy. It usually eases up after about 12 weeks and may be Nature's way of getting you to slow down until your pregnancy is firmly established. Practise relaxation with slow, gentle breathing, and avoid changing position too quickly. Many women find it helpful to sip milk or nibble dry biscuits, to give something for the stomach to work on between meals.

• **I get a lot of heartburn. What can I do apart from take medicine?**
Avoid rich or spicy foods and large meals. Keep putting bland food, such as a dry biscuit, into your stomach to absorb excess gastric juices. Watch your posture to avoid compression around the waist. Focus on the diaphragm and breathe deeply rather than in the upper chest only. Lean back from the waist with your palms pressed against your lumbar spine.

• **I feel sleepy, lethargic and tired most of the time. Any suggestions?**
This is Nature's way of getting you to rest, and the cure is to do so. Prioritize your activities and cut out the least essential ones to create more space in your life. Establishing a pregnancy takes up a great deal of energy but the good news is that you are likely to feel full of vitality once this early stage has passed.

• **Pregnancy is a totally new experience for me and I am really worried that I may miscarry.**
Breathe deeply and foster feelings of contentment and trust in Nature. Remember that your baby is becoming more firmly established in your body with every week that passes. Trust in the whole process, nurture your mind and body and enjoy regular relaxation practices – stresses of any kind will only increase any chance of miscarriage.

• **I feel anxious because I do not know how to cope with my pregnancy or if I'll be able to cope with my baby when he or she arrives.**
This problem arises because we can feel isolated in modern society. Many of us do not have an extended family on hand to support and advise us through the important stages in our lives, as would have been the case in past generations.

Help and reassurance are available, however. Join an antenatal group and make friends with other mothers-to-be – preferably in your neighbourhood, so you can easily get together to share experiences. Get to know women with babies and children and handle their babies, so that you will feel more confident when your own baby arrives. Joining a special prenatal yoga class or group gives women a regular opportunity to relax and become stronger and more confident. Above all, concentrate on breathing, relaxing – and trusting your inner wisdom.

15–30
weeks

Your pregnancy is now firmly
established and you should be feeling
full of vigour and joy, especially if you
have been practising yoga regularly
along the lines suggested so far. It is
time to focus on building up strength
and stamina, on making space to
"breathe for two" as your baby grows,
and on creating and maintaining the
best possible alignment of the spine at
all times. Most of all – time to enjoy
your pregnancy.

breathing for two

You are likely to be feeling much more energetic during this middle stage, so enjoy your vitality – many of the yoga routines designed for these months are lively, invigorating, almost dance-like. They get your breathing and circulation working optimally and the vigorous arm movements and upward stretches, plus deep breathing, help blood circulate through the abdominal organs and bring fresh, nourishing blood to your baby via the placenta.

You will find at this stage that your balance changes as your abdomen enlarges, so it is important to take your centre of gravity downward, while keeping your spine stretched up and your chest open. This upright, graceful stance will make you feel elegant and confident and also allows more space to be created around the diaphragm, which needs to find room to contract downward so that you are able to breathe really deeply and fully.

"Oneness of breath and mind... this is called Yoga, integration."

Maitri Upanishad 25

31 Sunwheel stretch

This exercise really focuses on upper body stretches to open the chest and loosen the shoulders. The movements wake up the whole of the upper spine and dissolve tightness in the neck, shoulders and arms – this is particularly helpful if you spend a lot of time sitting at a desk or driving a car. These movements also create more space in the abdomen, so that your digestive system has room to function and your baby has room to grow.

▷ **1** Sit with knees a comfortable width apart and feet firmly planted on the floor. Tuck your coccyx under so that your pelvis is level – imagine that the pelvis is a bowl of water and you don't want to spill any of it. Stretch up through your spine from the base to the crown, with your neck long and shoulders relaxed and down. Breathe in deeply to open and lift the chest. Hold the lift as you breathe out, drawing your shoulder blades together with arms relaxed and then pushing the palms down toward the floor with fingers spread wide, to end with straight arms. Repeat, pushing down against imaginary resistance with each breath out and relaxing as you breathe in.

△ **2** Repeat, but this time start with your elbows bent and hands pointing up as you breathe in – this is so that you create a greater push downward as you breathe out. Make your movements graceful and rhythmical, rather like a seated dance.

△ **3** Then, on each breath out, push strongly away from you to the sides, with your palms at shoulder level (the picture shows mid-push; you finish the push with straight arms). Engage the muscles around your spine and the back of your waist as you push. Relax as you breathe in. Repeat.

△ **4** On an out breath, stretch your palms to the sides with arms raised as high as you can, engaging your upper arms and back muscles. Finally, repeat the arm movements in reverse order, moving down until your arms are beside you. Repeat the whole sequence several times.

32 Swing high, swing low

This movement should be done rhythmically and with enthusiasm. It loosens up all the joints from your heels to your fingertips and blows away the cobwebs from your mind.

◁ **1** Stand with feet comfortably apart and knees well bent, and rotate your upper body from side to side, making sure your arms are loose and relaxed. Keep your spine upright, your hips and legs steady and your centre of gravity low.

◁ **2** Now stretch your arms right up to the right and clap your hands. Then sink into the previous position before stretching up to the left to clap your hands. Keep breathing deeply and vigorously as you alternately sink and relax then stretch to each side in turn.

33 Centring down

Getting your legs, rather than your lower back, to support your increasing weight and bulk is probably the most important postural adjustment that you can make during your pregnancy because it will save you from backache. Your womb is situated in the lower abdomen, which is held in place by the spine at the back, the pelvic girdle below and the hips on each side, so it has nowhere to expand as your baby grows except upward and forward. Any upward growth is constrained by your digestive organs and diaphragm, so most of the bulk has to move forward. This extra weight should flow downward through strong and well-toned legs, restoring your vital balance and centre of gravity.

△ **1** Stand with legs apart, feet firmly planted and knees loose. Stretch your spine upwards, taking your weight downwards through your legs. Press your palms together at throat height with elbows out to the sides. Breathe in and expand the lungs at the back by opening your back ribs more.

△ **2** As you breathe out stretch your arms forward and bend deeply at the knees. Hold a moment, then breathe in again. Repeat often.

Yoga and movement

When you are pregnant it is better to move through a variety of yogic positions, in a type of yogic dance, than to hold each position separately. This encourages deeper breathing, which is important as your breath provides oxygen for your baby's metabolism as well as your own. The yogic dance creates more flexibility in all your joints, making you feel loose and limber despite the added weight and bulk of your growing baby. Moving the spine rhythmically in all directions takes pressure off the lower back and strengthens all the muscles that hold the spine in alignment. Moving with knees well bent ensures that you avoid arching your back and that your spine and pelvis remain perfectly aligned. Your shoulders and neck should remain relaxed throughout.

34 Pat on the back

This free and rhythmic swinging movement loosens the tensions that so readily gather around the upper spine and shoulders after sitting. It also eases stresses in the joints of the hands and arms.

△ 1 Stand tall, with knees loose and coccyx tucked under. Swing your upper body from the shoulders, letting your arms and hands hang freely. Swing from one side to the other, but face to the front – your head and hips do not move.

△ 2 Repeat this relaxed swinging movement, but this time bend your elbows so you bring one hand right up and slightly over your shoulder, as though patting yourself on the back, and the other arm around to the back of your waist.

35 Ball of energy (1)

Imagine that you are playing with a huge, soft, invisible ball of energy. You create it by rubbing your palms briskly together, rather like rubbing two sticks together to create a flame. Then separate your hands a little before bringing them closer together in a pumping or kneading movement to enlarge your energy ball. Use your imagination and sense of touch, feeling that you are actually plumping up the ball of energy, tossing it from one hand to the other and holding it lightly between your fingertips as it grows and grows.

△ **1** Keeping your knees well bent and spine stretched, bend forward with your ball of energy, holding it lightly between your open palms.

△ **2** Now toss the invisible ball of energy to the side, twisting your body in a wide movement, but without moving your feet at all.

△ **3** Catch the ball above your head, with both arms. Keep your arms and legs slightly bent, and feel that you are centred around the naval area.

△ **4** Compress your ball, then roll it across your body, first on one side then on the other, twisting your body in a wide movement, from a strong base.

△ **5** Now expand the ball of energy, holding it with your arms wide to the sides and opening your chest. Your base should be strong, with knees slightly bent.

△ **6** Be inventive and lively as you continue to play with the ball, stretching and moving in all directions. When you have done enough, hold it between your palms and squeeze it smaller and smaller until it disappears between your palms.

Gentle twists and shoulder stretches

Vigorous exercise with arm movements and deep, natural breathing is a good way of keeping healthy, strong and supple while you are carrying your baby. It gets your circulation going, makes you feel great and relieves any strain, tension and tiredness that may have been building up in your neck and shoulders. It also exercises the muscles of the trunk and spine. These kinds of invigorating movements require both concentration and focus. They are most effective if you keep your knees bent throughout.

36 Thunder claps

These positions work the muscles across the chest and upper spine to lift the sternum and open the chest for deeper breathing, as well as opening and rotating the shoulder joints and strengthening the arms to relieve stiffness and tension. The pectoral muscles across the upper chest can become shortened if we slouch forward, especially when sitting at a desk or table and leaning upon our elbows. Let the vigorous rhythm of this exercise do the stretching for you, even if you can't clap behind your back at first. You will soon loosen up with frequent practice and enjoy the feeling of openness in the chest.

◁ **1** Stand tall through your spine, but with knees well bent and feet more than hip-width apart. Stretch your arms out to the front and clap your hands at shoulder level, reaching forward to open the back of the shoulders without moving the spine.

◁ **2** Now take your hands behind you and as high up as you can, to open the shoulder joints at the front and stretch the pectoral muscles across the upper chest. Bring your palms together to clap, straightening your arms if you can.

37 Disco twist

This is a rhythmic, twisting movement done with feet wide and knees well bent. Get into the swing of it, following your natural rhythm, and really get your breath and bloodstream moving. Stop as soon as you feel out of breath and rest in the starting position before moving on to the next exercise.

◁ **1** Stand with knees springy and loose and feet comfortably apart, arms relaxed.

◁ **2** Lift your chest and twist your upper body to the left, and also swing your arms and hands to the left. Bend your knees a little more to dip to the left, lift up again and twist to the right and repeat. Keep your coccyx tucked under, your spine upright and your legs springy as you twist from one side to the other.

38 Crossovers

These wide, sweeping movements combine stretching with a bending and twisting of the trunk. They require mental focus and deep, rhythmical breathing, and will fill you with energy, so practise them regularly. Circle your arms boldly, as though they have flags attached and you want to be seen from a distance. Crossovers require good co-ordination and are best done naturally and vigorously, without too much thought.

Start out by doing the sequence as a plain twist-and-stretch, feeling the lengthening in each side of your body as you alternate arms. Then build up to a much more fluid, wider circling movement, by stretching up higher, bending lower at the knees and twisting more deeply. Eventually, you should feel that as soon as you reach the maximum stretch on one arm, the other arm is sinking down to create another circle overlapping the previous one.

△ **1** Stand with knees springy and loose and feet a comfortable width apart – as you did in Step 1 of the Disco Twist (37).

△ **2** Slowly twist the upper body to the left as you raise your right arm in front of you and stretch it up high. Look up at it.

△ **3** Start to twist to the right as you start to lower your right arm in a circle behind you. Keep the chest open and your knees bent. At the same time start to take your left arm in front of you.

△ **4** When your left arm is stretched right up, look at your left hand. Try to make as straight a line as possible from your back heel to the very tip of the middle finger of your stretched hand.

△ **5** Lower your left arm behind you as you twist to the left. Bring your right arm to the front and across your body, ready to raise it again to complete the double circle. Repeat several times.

The three movements of the pelvis

Flexibility in the pelvis is natural in young children, and also in adults who live in traditional societies without the comforts and technology that we take for granted. But our sophisticated, Western way of life inhibits this flexibility, from schooldays onwards. We don't squat down to wash clothes or prepare food. Instead, we spend most of our waking hours in one form of chair or another while we chat, read, use the computer, and even while travelling. In order to regain our innate grace and suppleness, and to maintain it throughout our lives, we need to relearn the natural ways of holding and moving our bodies. Flexibility in the spine, hips and pelvis is especially important during pregnancy, as it alleviates many common discomforts, such as backache, sciatica and cramps, and also prepares the body for active, easy birthing.

"How long will you keep expecting answers from outside? Just go inside."

Frederick Leboyer

39 Seated pelvic rolls

Your lower abdominal muscles and the long transverse abdominal muscles (at the sides of the trunk) need to be strong and active, or they fail to play their part in supporting the weight of the body and leave your lower back muscles to carry the whole load. This exercise is a good way of strengthening both these sets of muscles.

△ **1** Sit squarely in a sturdy, upright chair, facing the back of the chair. Place your sitting bones near the front of the seat and hold on to the back of the chair for support. Arch your lower back strongly, lowering the front rim of your pelvis forward and bringing your abdomen closer to the chair. Feel the muscles of your spine contracting strongly as the abdominal muscles relax.

△ **2** Reverse this movement by tilting your pelvis back to lift the front rim of the pelvis. Stretch and relax your lower spine. The lower abdominal muscles are now contracting strongly.

△ **3** Now contract the long muscles on your right side, while consciously relaxing and stretching the ones on the left. This will lift your right hip up toward your right ribs, so that you are sitting on one side of the lower pelvis (your left sitting bone). Repeat this on the other side. Gradually combine these movements into a flowing, clockwise roll. Then repeat in an anti-clockwise direction.

40 Standing pelvic roll

This is a stronger, standing version of Seated Pelvic Rolls (39). It can be practised easily in any spare moment. If the abdomen feels distended and crowded by the growing baby, a few pelvic rolls can quickly create more space and relieve uncomfortable pressure. Placing your hands on your hips helps you to focus on the pelvic girdle and become more aware of its range of movement.

△ **1** Stand with feet apart, knees bent and springy. Place your hands on the front of your hip bones. Keep your whole spine stretched up from the base and through your neck and shoulders to the crown. Tilt your pelvis up on the left side so that you contract the transverse abdominal muscles on the left side and relax them on the right side. Don't move above the waist.

△ **2** Now drop your pelvis on the left side and tilt it up on the right side. Practise these two movements until they are smooth and flowing.

△ **3** Stand up straight again and roll the rim of the pelvis forward and upward, tucking your coccyx under and lengthening and relaxing through your lower spine. Avoid clenching your buttocks, as you allow the lower abdominal muscles to stretch with the forward movement.

△ **4** Tilt the rim of your pelvis down and back to arch your lower back. These four movements make up the pelvic roll. Continue round clockwise – left hip up, pelvic rim up, right hip up, pelvic rim down – in a smooth, rolling movement. Finish with the same number of anti-clockwise rolls.

41 Jump for joy

This is an exuberant movement, celebrating the lightness and grace in your legs and hips. Feel yourself bursting with energy and full of the joys of life as you open your hips and chest wide, affirming your trust in a world that welcomes the baby that you are now carrying within you. You can even include a light jump in the air if you feel like it.

△ **1** Stand on your right leg, keeping your right knee relaxed. As you raise your left knee in front of you to hip height, bring your elbows high and wide, with the backs of your hands above your face.

△ **2** Open your left hip to swing your left knee to the side at hip height, flinging your arms wide at shoulder height. Step down on to your left side and bring your right knee up to repeat on the other side. Keep your arms circling.

Gaining strength and stamina

The following movements have isometric qualities: that is, one set of muscles contracts strongly to push against a second set that are resisting the push. The result, with practice, is that both sets of muscles get stronger by pushing against each other. There is also a centring and stabilizing effect, as the two-way push ripples throughout the whole body. Each strong pushing movement should be balanced by a letting-go pose, so that muscular strength is built up rather than muscular tension. Isometric exercise helps posture, breathing and spinal alignment. It builds strength symmetrically, which is especially important during pregnancy.

42 Swing and release

In this vigorous exercise, the palms are pressed firmly together to strengthen the muscles of the hands and arms, and especially the muscles that lie each side of the upper spine. Strength here makes it easy to maintain a good upright posture through the spine and neck, so that the circulation of the blood and the messages passing along the nervous system can flow freely through the neck and trunk. Raising the arms while pressing the hands together strengthens the muscles at the sides of the body and lifts the sternum for deeper breathing.

◁ 1 Stand with your feet a comfortable width apart and your knees bent but relaxed and loose. Bring your palms together and bend forward from the hips so that your fingertips touch the floor. Breathe out in this position.

△ 2 Stretch your arms forward, pushing the palms hard against each other and engaging the muscles of your upper back for lifting. Breathe in strongly, raising your head, arms and trunk up and to the right side, twisting the spine to the right from the waist. Hold this position for a few seconds, pressing your palms together and feeling your muscles along your arms and spine.

△ 3 On a strong breath out through the mouth in a "HAH" sound, drop back to your starting position, knees well bent. Keep your hands together and strong, like a knife slicing through bread. Let go of all effort as you breathe in and out to relax in the starting position. Breathe in again strongly to repeat the upward stretch and pushing movements to the left side. Repeat a few times.

43 Push and release

Here, two different isometric pushing movements are counterbalanced by the same open and surrendering pose. This is an important principle in everyday life as well as in yoga practice. We should always relax between activities in order to dissolve any physical, emotional or mental tensions before they can take a hold. In this way we build up our strength and stamina rather than depleting our reserves.

△ **1** Stand with your spine erect, coccyx tucked under, pelvis level and knees well bent. Clasp your hands at chest level and push one hand hard against the other for two strong breaths in and out.

△ **2** Breathe in, then, with a voiced-out breath "aaah", open your arms to the side in a surrendering gesture. Keep the chest open and the back straight. Rest in this position and take a deep breath, relaxing the facial muscles.

△ **3** Bring your arms straight out in front of you and make fists. Push your fists forward, opening and stretching your back and maintaining balance by using your lower abdominal and front thigh muscles. Then relax as before in the surrender position. Repeat several times.

44 Hip openers in pairs

Two people exercising together can be good fun, but you will also help each other to develop strength and stamina and to improve muscle tone. Be careful to judge your partner's strength and balance – it is easier to work with a partner who is roughly the same height and weight as you are. Some of these positions can also be practised on your own, by using a wall to lean against or a strong counter to pull on.

▷ **1** Stand facing each other with feet planted firmly, quite wide apart, and knees loosely bent. Take hold of each other's forearms with a firm grip. Both partners then bend forward at the waist. Adjust your position so that each partner makes a right angle with their legs and trunk. Once settled, start to pull away from each other. Stretch the base of your spine and make space in the lumbar region, wriggling your hips from side to side.

◁ **2** Face to face and gripping each other's forearms, both partners lift their left knees out to the side, opening up the hip joints. This mutual support helps you to keep your balance and also allows you to extend the raised knee further out and back than you could on your own.

▷ **3** After extending the raised knees as far back as possible, both partners land their left foot softly on the floor behind them. Raise the left leg again for another round and repeat a few times. Now

kneeling stretches

Some kneeling positions enable you to build up strength and stamina (to help you carry your baby without getting tired), and kneeling stretches can prevent and ease low back pain. At the same time, kneeling exercises focus upon the birthing muscles. The latter is especially important if this is your first baby, as these muscles will not have been used before. Getting used to a kneeling position for your stretches is an important part of preparing for labour, since many women prefer this position in childbirth.

45 Cat pose

The Cat Pose is traditionally used to loosen all the joints before going into classical yogic seated poses. A simpler version, called the "kitten roll" here, is included as a warm-up. Avoid sagging at the waist by holding your middle spine firmly in line, like a table top, as you move through the rolls.

▷ **1** Kneel on your yoga mat with knees about hip-width apart, so that there is plenty of room for your baby. Place cushions under your knees, if you like. Sit back on your heels and, without lifting your buttocks, stretch your arms out in front, about shoulder-width apart. Crawl forward with your fingers, anchoring your buttocks on to your heels. Feel the stretch through your spine and breathe slowly into it to loosen tension in your back, hips or shoulders.

△ **2** For the "kitten roll", sit back on your heels before breathing in to bring your weight forward on to your elbows. Lift your shoulders as you breathe out to arch your spine and tuck your coccyx under before rolling back on to your heels. Repeat the roll several times, and as you do so, focus your attention on feeling the stretch at the back of your waist.

△ **3** For the "cat roll", bring your weight forward on to spread palms as you breathe in, so your shoulders are directly above your wrists, your arms are straight but not locked at the elbow and your back is flat. This is the classic Cat Pose. Breathe out to arch and stretch your spine before sitting back on your heels, without moving your hands. Breathe in to repeat the rolling movement.

46 Hip and knee circles

These circles are practised while in the Cat Pose (45). They loosen tightness in the hip joints, can relieve cramps in the groin and increase the circulation of blood around the abdomen and pelvis.

▷ Place yourself in the Cat Pose (45), with your weight evenly distributed and your back and head held firmly in line. Raise your right knee from the floor, keeping it bent at a right angle, and move it around in small circles parallel to the floor so that you are rotating the hip joint. After circling clockwise and

47 Shoulder and elbow circles

These circles are great for relieving tension in the neck and shoulders, stretching the pectoral muscles and opening the chest for deeper breathing. Both exercise 46 and this exercise provide the same benefits as swimming movements.

△ **1** Place yourself in the Cat Pose (45) and then sit back on your heels. Keeping your weight evenly balanced, and your spine and head firmly in line, stretch your right arm out in front of you.

△ **2** Bend your right elbow and bring your arm up and back in a circle, turning your head and opening the right side of your chest and shoulder. Lift the elbow as high as you can before stretching the arm to the front. Repeat on the left.

48 Tiger stretch and relax (1)

This is one of the best ways to relieve lower backache and sciatica. This can sometimes become a problem as your pregnancy advances and the weight of your baby presses on the sciatic nerve as it emerges from the lower spine and carries on down your leg. You will need to balance firmly on strong wrists and hands as you raise your leg parallel to the floor.

△ **1** Place yourself in the Cat Pose (45) with spine stretched and firm, especially at the waist. Slowly raise your right leg behind you until it is parallel to the floor, neither higher nor lower. Stretch right through your leg and into your toes, and kick away any tension or pressure.

△ **2** Let your leg sink limply to the floor and relax it completely. Maintain your balance and the strength in your spine, but drop your right hip. Shake your leg loosely from hip to toes to release cramps or pressure on the sciatic nerve. Then readjust your position and do the same movements with the left leg.

49 Manual back stretch

As your baby grows it becomes ever more important to relax frequently and to ease away tiredness and tension. A partner or friend can work wonders, simply by gently helping your spine to stretch as you lie comfortably draped over a beanbag or pillows, either on your bed or on the floor. Your helper does not need to be an expert, just intuitive and happy to be guided by you to discover the position where you can relax and breathe most deeply.

▷ Your helper needs to be in a firm, comfortable position, where they do not strain their own back. He or she extends their hands so their fingers trace light pressure either side of your spine as you breathe out. They release pressure on each in breath. Your partner should avoid direct pressure on the spine and check what feels best for you. The aim is to reduce compression

Your birthing muscles

A sphincter is a ring-shaped muscle that acts like a valve by squeezing tightly around the bottom of a tube to keep the contents in. If you want to release the contents, you simply relax the sphincter muscle, or you can get it to push the contents out by controlling the flow with rhythmic pulses. Women have three "tubes" that are either sphincters or are sphincter-like. These open at the base of the body – an area often called the pelvic floor – through the perineum (a mass of muscle that stretches right across the base of the body and holds the abdomen's contents in place.) Each of these openings is controlled by strong muscles, which are:

- the anal tube at the end of our digestive system, which opens to release waste matter. It is found near the base of the spine, at the back of the pelvic floor;
- the urethra – the tube leading from the bladder. This is found close to the pubic bone, at the front of the pelvic floor;
- the muscles each side of the vagina, which can contract and release around the cervix. The cervix thins out during labour to become the birth canal and let your baby descend through the vagina. Squeezing the vaginal muscles – "pulling up inside" – helps you locate and feel your cervix.

With regular practice, you can learn to contract or relax these muscles at will. This will help you throughout pregnancy (when your baby is pressing down against the pelvic floor), during the birth (to help control the baby's movement down through the birth canal), and after the birth (to restore perineal muscle tone as quickly as possible, thus avoiding many common postnatal problems).

exercising the birthing muscles

Yogic philosophy maintains that energy follows thought. So focusing on muscle groups that we usually ignore helps to bring movement to the area and encourages awareness, which leads in turn to control of those muscles. Using the breath intensifies

THE BIRTHING MUSCLES

The pelvic area at around mid-term
Note how the baby presses against the internal organs shown

spine

uterus

cervix

bladder

pelvic floor
urethra

vagina

rectum

anal sphincter
muscles

anus

front of body

The perineum
(seen from below)

**The red, striated areas
are muscle**

clitoris
urethra
vagina

anus

gluteus
maximus

back of body

the muscular action. Yogic actions are never mechanical because you are using your breath and awareness simultaneously with the contraction and relaxation of the muscles. By connecting breath with muscular action you are toning, in a unique way, the muscles of the perineum, including those that attach it to the pelvis at the front and the lower spine at the back.

Begin your birthing muscle workout with the anal sphincter, contracting and

releasing it in turn. Focus on how this feels, so that you learn to draw in the anus on a breath in and slowly release it on a breath out. Now focus on the sphincter of the urethra, squeezing it in and relaxing it in small, rapid movements. Finally, focus on the vaginal muscles, squeezing them tightly to draw your pelvic floor up and in. You will find that the lower abdomen is also drawn up and inward. These are the "birthing muscles" that you want to strengthen.

50 Pelvic floor stretches

In this modification of the Cat Pose (45) your weight is distributed through your knees and elbows, leaving your lower back and pelvis weightless, released from the constraints of gravity that usually restrict flexibility in this area.

◁ **1** Kneel in the Cat Pose (45), with your knees spread wide enough to accommodate your baby as you lean forward on to your elbows. Place your head on a cushion if it is more comfortable. Distribute your weight evenly between your elbows and your knees, so that your head and neck are comfortable and your coccyx is raised as high as possible. Focus upon your pelvic floor, then exercise the three main birthing "sphincters" one by one, as explained on the opposite page.

◁ **2** Alternate the kneeling position with this pelvic lift, which uses different sets of inner muscles. Lie on your back with your buttocks on a cushion to raise the pelvis. Keep your knees bent, with feet apart and firmly planted on the floor. Place your hands over your baby to feel the movement as you squeeze the whole pelvic floor in and up. Hold the squeeze for a few breaths to strengthen these muscles, then let go and relax completely. Repeat several times.

51 Supported pelvic floor lift

Your baby needs space to pass down through the vagina. This space is created naturally, as hormones are released during pregnancy to loosen the ligaments that hold your bones in place. This allows your pelvic opening to widen naturally. You can help by relaxing your hip and leg muscles in a wide-legged seated position, reclining comfortably against a beanbag or other support. Do not force yourself, just breathe gently in this position. Once the muscles around the groin have gently relaxed, the ligaments can stretch. In addition, the more relaxed you are the easier it is to practise strengthening the inner muscles of the perineum and vagina.

△ **1** Sit with your legs as wide apart as is comfortable for you. Make sure that your spine is well supported, especially at the base. Flex your ankles and stretch through your legs. Lean back and relax. The muscles around the groin area should be especially relaxed, to allow the ligaments to stretch.

△ **2** Now clasp your hands in front of you at chest height, breathing in as you press your palms firmly together, and at the same time contract the muscles of the perineum and vagina. Hold this contraction for a breath or two, and then relax completely before repeating.

seated stretches

These easy stretches can be done at any time, sitting on a chair or on the floor with your back upright and legs uncrossed. The more you practise, the more flexible and relaxed your whole body will become. If you have to spend hours in front of a computer or driving, for example, try to stretch regularly. You should, of course, be working your inner muscles in the lower abdominal and pelvic area while seated throughout the day. One of the skills that comes with regular yoga practice is the ability to work one area of the body quite strongly while keeping all the other parts completely relaxed.

52 Neck rolls

Tension is apt to build up around the neck and shoulders when you sit and concentrate for any length of time, whether travelling or working at a desk. You can prevent this build-up by being aware of your posture, and by stopping for a short break whenever you can.

▷ Sit erect on an upright chair, maintaining the stretch through your spine as you relax your arms and shoulders. Sit with knees wide and feet firmly on the floor, resting your hands comfortably on your thighs. Relax your neck muscles and bring your chin forward, lengthening the back of your neck, then round to your right shoulder. Bring your chin forward again then round to your left shoulder. Repeat gently, with relaxed breathing.

53 Chest expander

This energizing exercise strengthens the muscles that hold your upper spine in place, so it is excellent for improving your posture, as well as increasing your lung capacity for deeper breathing. Try it when you are feeling mentally tired.

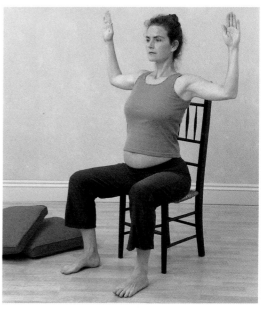

△ **1** Sit upright, with knees wide and feet firmly planted on the floor. Raise your elbows to shoulder height. As you breathe out press your forearms and palms together in front of your face.

△ **2** As you breathe in take your elbows high and back, squeeze your shoulder blades together, lifting your sternum and stretching your pectoral muscles across your upper chest. Bring the elbows forward again. Repeat several times.

54 Seated side stretch

This exercise prevents and alleviates heartburn. It opens the sides of the body to make more room in the abdomen for better functioning of the diaphragm and the digestive organs. It also gives your developing baby more room to move around. Sit on a firm chair with knees wide and feet on the floor.

◁ 1 Bring your left arm out to the side and up overhead, stretching your whole left side. Resting your right elbow on your right thigh, turn your head to look up at your outstretched hand and breathe deeply into the stretched side, holding the position. Repeat on the other side.

▷ 2 For a stronger stretch, place your right ankle on your left thigh then raise your right arm. Hold your foot with your left hand, ankle flexed and in line as you drop your right knee to the side. Stretch your right arm up. Hold, breathing deeply. Repeat on the other side.

55 Seated stretches in pairs

This lively sequence is fun to do and really gets your energy flowing and blood circulation moving. If you are different heights, then the shorter partner can sit on a cushion to even things out.

△ 1 Sit back to back legs crossed and spines pulled upward. Lean on each other to increase awareness of the position of your spines, and adjust your alignment. Breathe deeply and notice how you start to breathe together.

△ 2 Face each other with right legs straight and left knees bent (left feet against right thighs). Sit up tall with your palms pressed against your partner's palms. Circle your hands out to the sides and in again. Change legs and repeat.

△ 3 Keep in the same position, but this time both partners use isometric pressure on each other's palms to rotate the trunk, twisting first to one side and then the other. Look over your shoulder to take the twist through your upper spine and neck.

△ 4 Sit back to back with your legs crossed or knees comfortably bent. Link arms and rock back and forth, so that one partner folds forward as the other stretches backward. Keep your spines in contact while rocking.

△ 5 Hold each other's hands, then stretch your arms out to the sides and up overhead to maintain a stretch in the sides of your trunk. Go gently and learn to sense what the other person needs – no force, pulling or pushing.

lying down stretches

When you are tired – or after your standing, kneeling and sitting exercises – you can lie down to relax and also stretch, so that you are still gaining strength and flexibility while the floor supports the weight of your baby. You will feel much more renewed and refreshed after these kinds of gentle movements than if you were simply to collapse in a heap in front of the television. Remember to keep a large cushion handy beside you – for total relaxation after you have completed the stretches.

56 Side loosener

In these movements, the lower side of the trunk (the side that is lying against the floor) is gently stretched and the upper side is strongly contracted. You need to avoid overbalancing on to your back as you raise your upper leg, as this will reduce the contraction of the transverse abdominal muscles.

CAUTION
It is safe to lie on your back for the first 30 or so weeks of pregnancy, provided you feel comfortable. After this time, always recline or lie on your side for both stretching and relaxing. This avoids pressure on the main blood vessels to and from the uterus.

△ **1** Lie on your left side with your left knee bent (your other leg outstretched but still relaxed) and your left arm outstretched under your head. Place your right hand on the floor in front of you to help you maintain your balance. Lean forward as you raise your bent right knee and bring it toward your elbow.

△ **2** Make gentle circles with the right knee, opening up your right groin and leg to extend your right leg slightly behind you. Do not over-stretch yourself. Return to the start position with your right knee bent and repeat the movement. If you are skipping step 3, roll on to your right side and repeat with the left leg.

△ **3** This is an optional extra step, if it feels comfortable and enjoyable. If you have been circling the right leg, stretch this leg straight up, ankle flexed, to open the right hip. Press forward into your right hand to avoid rolling backwards. Hold the stretch, feeling the muscles in your right side contract.

△ **4** At the end of a series of leg-stretches, relax for a few moments, placing the cushion between your knees to take the pressure off your lower abdomen.

57 Pelvic lift

In this position, you contract and strengthen the muscles around the base of your spine and make space at the front of your body. It is an excellent position for focusing on breathing deeply because you use all your abdominal muscles while the chest muscles are held open and immobile. It is also an excellent position for pulling your inner muscles in and up to strengthen the pelvic floor muscles in relation to the muscles of the abdomen and back.

◁ **1** Lie on your back on the floor, with your head on a cushion if this feels more comfortable. Bend your knees and plant your feet on the floor more than hip-width apart. Turn your toes slightly inward to engage the muscles of the inner thighs and groin area. Place your arms alongside your body with the palms down. Now breathe in.

◁ **2** Breathe out as you lift your pelvis from the floor, engaging your perineal muscles and tucking your coccyx under to extend your lower back. Breathe in, continuing to lift your pelvis by contracting the muscles behind your waist and in your upper back. Breathe deeply in this position, focusing on your diaphragm muscle. Then lower your spine slowly to the floor, vertebra by vertebra from the neck downward. Rest and repeat several times.

◁ **3** Lie on your back with a cushion under the small of your back. Stretch your legs out at least hip-width apart and place your hands around your baby. Close your eyes and relax deeply for a few minutes.

58 Double cycling

This isometric exercise strengthens the muscles in your feet, legs, hips and pelvis as you push your feet against those of your partner.

▷ Lie on your back on the floor, supporting your upper body on your elbows and forearms. Place your soles against your partner's soles and push against them as though riding a bicycle. For each person, one leg pushes forward against your partner as the other leg is being pushed back by your partner.

Changing positions in pregnancy

As the weight in your abdomen increases, it becomes more tiring to do certain everyday movements, such as rising from a chair or getting out of bed in the morning. This is inevitable, but there is no need to struggle if you learn some simple steps, preferably before you need them. As your baby grows in your womb (and also after the birth), you will be glad of your strong leg and arm muscles, as well as your strong back. Here's how to make these movements gracefully and easily.

59 Standing from sitting

It is more difficult to haul yourself out of a chair if you are slumped or sprawled backwards. Let your muscles hold your body firmly, so that gravity becomes your friend rather than your enemy. Of course, it is also easier to rise lightly from a firm, upright chair than a soft, low sofa, so choose carefully where you sit as well as how.

◁ **1** First sit up straight, so that your weight passes in a straight line from your head, through your neck and into your spine. Place your feet apart and firmly planted on the floor, ready to receive your weight. Raise your elbows to lift up through your spine and chest. Keep the stretch.

◁ **2** Lean forward with your back straight and place your hands on your thighs. The thighs are among the strongest muscles in your body, designed for weight-bearing, so use them fully to protect your lower back. Press hard on your thighs with your arms.

△ **3** Rise gracefully and realign your spine before moving away from the chair.

60 Rolling out of bed

To begin this movement, make sure that you are lying facing the edge of the bed. You may like to rest or sleep with a cushion between your bent knees as this takes the pressure off your lower back and frees sensitive nerves in your back (particularly the sciatic nerve).

▷ **1** Lie on your side near the edge. You should have your lower elbow bent and your chest open – the ideal sleeping position for later pregnancy.

△ **2** To get up, roll more on to your front. Bring your top hand and your top knee over to the edge of the bed.

△ **3** Put your weight on your top hand, lifting your upper body, and slide your top leg over the edge of the bed to place your foot firmly on the floor. Raise your buttocks and rise out of bed.

61 Standing from lying

This technique will serve you well every time you get off your yoga mat after doing floor stretches or deep relaxation.

△ **1** Bend both knees and place your feet on the floor. Bring your right elbow to your left knee at about waist level.

△ **2** Roll on to your left hip, leaning on your bent left leg, and support your body on your right hand. Bring the left hand up to shoulder level too.

△ **3** Move on to all fours in the Cat Pose (45) and turn your toes under.

△ **4** Walk your hands back to your knees. Your knees will then come up from the floor as your weight shifts back, so that you are in a squatting position, with your heels as low as possible.

▷ **5** Engage your thigh muscles and rise slowly.

Some subtle yoga movements

Now for something totally different. You have discovered how effectively yoga helps you to strengthen your body and increase your awareness, and how you can use these benefits in your everyday life. Well, in yoga there are also certain positions that look – and are – simple to do, yet they create very subtle internal adjustments and strengthen groups of muscles that we are not usually aware of. These can bring huge benefits once you have explored, practised and become thoroughly familiar with them. These exercises require a calm, focused approach; in turn, they foster inner strength and self-confidence.

62 Gentle perineal stretch

This simple exercise should be done as often as possible from mid-pregnancy onwards, as it stretches all the muscles that make up the pelvic floor. It also strengthens, relaxes and brings awareness to the whole perineal area, which is the area through which your baby passes to be born. If the perineum is flexible, strong and lively, it helps you to give birth actively and with greater ease. You will be able to take your foot farther out to the side as you gradually loosen up with practice.

△ **1** From the Cat Pose (45), bring your left foot forward, placing it as far to the left of your hands as you can manage. Lean forward and breathe in deeply, keeping your spine stretched.

△ **2** Breathe out as you sit back on your right heel without moving your left foot. This stretches the perineal muscles. Repeat several times, then change sides and repeat.

63 Rib stretch with Namaste hand mudra

This powerful exercise helps you to open your lungs more fully and to breathe more deeply by stretching between the ribs, especially at the back where your ribs are attached to your spine. It brings increased awareness to your back and is also an isometric exercise that strengthens your arms and upper spinal muscles. A mudra is a gesture with a spiritual as well as a physical expression. Adding the Namaste Hand Mudra focuses your scattered thoughts and centres your vital energies. It should be practised frequently for greater posture awareness, increased vitality and a focused mind. In late pregnancy, this exercise helps to create more space in the chest for your lungs to expand as your baby develops below the diaphragm.

△ **1** Stand with your feet hip-width apart and knees loosely bent. Stretch the spine and drop the shoulders. Raise your elbows to the sides at shoulder height and press your palms together as you breathe in slowly and deeply. Feel your sternum rise and your ribs open at the back.

△ **2** Now, breathe out slowly as you bring your hands down, with palms still joined. Relax your chest completely. Pause and rest with the breath out, then repeat the sequence twice more. When you have finished, rest for a moment and observe how you feel deep inside.

64 Sectional breathing with mudras

You will probably be surprised to discover that your breathing changes according to the position of your hands in these subtle hand mudras. Ensure that the first three types of breathing come easily to you before you join them together in the complete yogic breath. Allow a minute or two of rest before and after this practice to gain maximum benefit.

◁ **1** Sit up straight with your chest lifted to make room for your breathing muscles to move freely. Place your hands at your lower abdomen with fingers pointing toward each other. Join the tips of your index fingers and thumbs together to create a closed circuit of energy. Breathe in deeply and feel your abdomen expand as your diaphragm contracts downward. This is called "lower breathing" and gives you energy. Breathe out and repeat.

◁ **2** Now change your hand position, so that your fingers are curled into your palms and your thumbs are free. Breathe in deeply and feel your sternum lift and your ribs move out to the sides. This is called "middle breathing" and it also gives you energy. It comes to your rescue when your growing baby makes it difficult for your diaphragm to contract downward fully. Breathe out and repeat.

◁ **3** Change your hand position again, so that your thumbs are enclosed within your curled fingers. Breathe in deeply and feel how your upper chest is now moving much more freely. This is called "upper breathing" and is very useful if you have indigestion. Breathe out and repeat. You may also need this during labour, so start practising now.

◁ **4** With your thumbs and fingers curled into your palms, press your knuckles together with the fingers of each hand back to back. Turn your palms upward, with your hands in front of you. Open your chest and breathe in fully, from the bottom of your lungs to the top. Breathe out fully and repeat several times. This is full yogic breathing, excellent for recharging your energy and integrating mind, body and spirit in the here and now.

balancing activity with relaxation

Our energy is called forth by stimulation, motivation, desire or need, which is the urge that gets us going every morning. Then we enjoy the experience of doing things and of being energetic, busy and involved. When this energy begins to ebb, we need to call it back within ourselves for recharging, so that we rest, relax and renew ourselves at every level by "just being".

If we are to maintain our zest for life, this cycle should be repeated throughout the day, until we finally wind down for our sleep at night. It is a rhythm as natural as breathing and it continues throughout life. Yet,

somehow, in our modern society, we have become addicted to just one phase of the cycle – the active phase – at the expense of the passive phase. We seem unable to respond to the need for rest even when we feel tired and depleted.

Yoga teaches us how to balance activity with rest, doing with being. It teaches us when and how to relax, and to respond to our body's signals that it is time for a short break. Deep relaxation does not take long and is less a question of time than of attitude. This vital life skill is one of yoga's most valuable gifts. First we become aware of the

rhythm of the breath and realize that each breath in is a muscular exertion; each breath out is the release that follows. Then we learn to apply this rhythm to all our activities – both mental and physical. We gradually learn to relax and release the toxins and tensions of living as they arise. It is their build-up that causes stress, congestion and poor functioning of body and mind.

With any relaxation practices, the most vital first step is to make yourself really comfortable, with support just where you need it, so that you can let all your muscles relax and your mind sink into repose.

65 Take your focus inward
"Time out" breaks work best when you have something gentle and non-stressful to focus on. Here are three useful suggestions.

◁ **1** It can be very soothing to just sit quietly and turn inward, becoming aware of your growing baby. Try focusing on your own gentle breathing or on feeling your baby's movement inside you.

△ **2** Gently massaging your wrists and all the little joints in your hands releases tension and helps to balance the nervous system and pelvic area.

△ **3** The same principle applies to massaging your inner ankles. This is the reflex area for your womb and massaging gently helps tone and strengthen.

66 Focus on your baby

By now your baby is probably moving around vigorously, alternating between periods of sleep and activity, and growing into a real person. Get to know this person who is coming into your life. Enjoy the communication of loving touch between you.

67 Focus on yourself

Being pregnant, and focusing on your baby, does not make you any less of a person yourself. Relax for your own well-being, too.

△ **1** Delight in noticing how your baby responds to the massaging movement of your hands.

△ **2** Take time to explore your baby's contours. Are those heels? Is that a head?

△ **3** Feel your breathing and your own glowing heart centre radiating outward. Just be.

68 Relax with your partner

Both of you should celebrate the experience of your pregnancy. Invest time in getting to know this new person who is coming into your lives. Touch and talk to your baby together.

▷ **1** Relax while your partner explores your baby's movements. By placing his hand right under the base of your uterus (thumbs on pubis, fingers extended out toward the hip bones), he can give you a strong resistance that deepens your breathing while relaxing – excellent preparation for breathing through contractions without over-tensing muscles.

▷ **2** In joint relaxation with your partner, you can both place your hands on the baby. This quiet communication through touch generates harmony between the three of you – now and into the future.

deep relaxation

Deep relaxation is an essential part of your yoga practice. It may come at the end of a daily yoga exercise and breathing session, if you have time, or you may find it more convenient to divide your yoga session into two parts. You may like to practise yoga exercises with short rests for breathing and relaxation in the morning, then add an extra half-hour slot for breathing and deep relaxation at another time of the day when you will not be disturbed. The more regular your practice, the better the results.

69 Modified positions for deep relaxation

As your baby grows, lying on your back will no longer be comfortable and, as it can restrict circulation, it is not a good idea. The classical yoga relaxation position needs to be modified from about 30 weeks onwards. You can bend your knees or place a cushion or blankets under your hips, lie on your side or lean forward over a beanbag. You can even relax deeply while sitting up, as long as you are well supported and your legs are not hanging down. Below are six alternatives for you to try.

> **CAUTION**
> Those with high blood pressure should not rest with arms raised above their head – it makes the heart work harder. It is fine to raise arms while exercising, as the blood is already moving briskly.

△ Place a firm cushion under the head, to lengthen the neck and stop the chin jutting up, and a soft one under waist and hips. With bent elbows, wrap your palms around the abdomen to keep contact with your baby.

△ Bend your knees out to the sides and bring the soles of your feet together. Place plenty of soft padding under the thighs and knees. This makes more space in the lower abdomen for your baby.

△ Place a beanbag under your legs and a cushion under the hips. Your raised legs improve blood flow to the heart and reduce swelling and aching legs; raised hips ease the lower back. This position can help turn a breech baby.

◁ Kneel down with knees wide, to allow plenty of room for your baby. Lean forward over a beanbag and rest your head in your arms. This is a very relaxing pose. The whole spine is gently stretched by the raised arms, the pelvis and hips are open, and the beanbag is taking the baby's weight.

▷ Push the beanbag against a wall for extra support and recline against it so that you are as comfortable as possible. Sit with your knees bent and out to the sides and add cushions underneath to open up your hips.

△ Lie on one side with a cushion between your knees and one under your head. Lying on your left side is a popular position as pregnancy advances, as it encourages the best presentation of the fetus for birth.

A sample mid-term practice

1

▷ **Swing and release (42)**

2

▽ **Supported pelvic floor lift (51)**

3

△ **Pelvic floor stretches (50)**

4

◁ **Sectional breathing with mudras (64)**

5

△ **Modified positions for deep relaxation (69)**

"The secret life stirs within me
O my darling, I can hear your
heartbeats."

Indian birth song

Questions and answers

• **I get a lot of backache, especially in my lower back.**
This is usually because of tightness (caused by tension) in the muscles of the lower back as well as weakness in the lower abdominal and pelvic floor muscles. Practise the movements suggested in this chapter to strengthen these groups of muscles so that they can help to support your spine and keep your trunk in good alignment.

• **I get pain in my groin or pelvis, which seems to be caused by pressure or constriction.**
This can be due to muscular weakness or imbalance causing poor posture and undue pressure from the growing baby in the pelvic area. Practise abdominal strengthening, as well as upper spine and arm movements that lift your chest and pull the weight of your baby upwards. When resting, keep your legs up and your hips raised, to ease any pressure.

• **The pressure of the baby on my bladder wakes me up at night and I have to keep getting up.**
Avoid drinking at bedtime, and sleep on your side with a pillow between your knees to take the pressure off your bladder.

• **My joints feel so loose that I am afraid they will not support my increasing weight.**
Hormones are released during pregnancy that soften the ligaments that hold your joints in place. This is to prepare the pelvic area to open and let your baby pass through the birth canal. Avoid overstretching in any position, especially in those joints that bear the body's weight, namely your hips, pelvis, lower back and knees.

• **I can't get a really good night's sleep, and this is making me feel so tired all of the time.**
This lack of sleep can be due to all kinds of things – such as pressure on your bladder, indigestion, or swelling and puffiness in your legs. Exercises that will help to ease these conditions are given throughout this chapter. It may also help to play your relaxation tape in bed, just before you go to sleep. When you wake in the night, focus on your breathing, commune with your baby and repeat the "seed thoughts" and affirmations that we talked about in the introduction. Provided that your mind is profoundly relaxed and peaceful you should not be deprived of the rest that you need, even if you are not actually asleep.

31+
weeks

During these last few weeks your priorities will be to keep yourself as fit and comfortable as possible, and to practise all the yoga techniques that can help you during the birthing process. These techniques prepare you physically, mentally and spiritually for labour, greatly empowering you from within. However your birthing may unfold, yoga will help you to feel centred and actively involved with your birth.

Yoga in late pregnancy

Your baby will be growing rapidly by now, so your yogic priorities need to change. First, you will need to protect your back much more by ensuring that your pelvic and leg muscles are able to carry the extra weight properly. Your focus will be on building power in these supporting muscles. This means paying more attention to centring and grounding exercises, and always remembering to keep your knees well bent in any of the standing poses and movements. Cushions and beanbags should be used to support your back at all times, to enable you to rest more deeply during relaxation. Secondly, you will need to make more space for your baby, your breathing and your digestive organs. Finally, you will be focusing specifically on increasing the tone in your birthing muscles – in other words, the muscles of your lower back, abdominal area and pelvic floor.

70 Centring into the earth

This exercise combines both power and release. Imagine that you are hauling yourself up a ladder, one arm at a time, and then climbing down again as you support your weight with your arms. Your legs should be well bent to support your weight. Feel a line of strength developing along a vertical axis between earth and sky, passing through your body.

△ **1** You are going to climb up your metaphorical ladder. Stand with knees bent and spine loose. Stretch first one arm overhead and then the other, as though you were climbing a rope ladder without your feet. Squeeze your fingers tightly to hold on to the ropes. When you get to the top, spend a few moments hanging from both arms, squeezing and releasing your hands.

△ **2** To climb down again, imagine you are going down a fireman's pole. All the strength is in your arms as you lower your weight one hand over the other down the pole. Slide down several times, bending your knees and grounding strongly along the vertical axis. These exercises can be done anytime, anywhere.

71 Supported side stretches

You need to practise side bending while sitting and resting your spine against a soft but firm support – here we show a beanbag placed against a wall, which is ideal.

▷ **1** Sit, leaning against a beanbag or a pile of cushions, with your legs stretched out in front of you and comfortably apart. Bring your hands behind your head with elbows wide and pressed back to open your chest and stretch the sides of your body – you can breathe much more deeply in this position. Relax as you lengthen the breath out.

△ **2** Still leaning back, tilt your upper trunk to one side as you breathe out. Breathe in to straighten up and then tilt to the other side as you breathe out again. Repeat a few times.

△ **3** Now, open your arms wide and stretch overhead, breathing deeply. This stretch really eases pressure in the lower body.

△ **4** Keep one arm overhead and take the other forearm on to your thigh for support, then tilt to the side on a breath out. Breathe in to straighten up and out to bend to the other side.

72 Hugging rest

This resting pose is ideal for late pregnancy. You may also find it comfortable for deep relaxation. The beanbag (or pile of cushions) supports your abdomen, spine and head. Spread your arms wide to lift and create more space in your chest.

◁ Kneel down, facing the beanbag, with your knees spread wide to accommodate your baby. Now rest the front of your body and the side of your face against the softness of the beanbag and give it a big hug. Breathe deeply and relax completely.

Light on your feet, light at heart

To say that you are light and full of vitality may sound like a counsel of perfection when you are carrying around a baby that is almost ready to be born. It is, however, largely an attitude of both mind and heart. At this stage of your pregnancy it is very helpful to think "strong" and "graceful" simply to be in harmony with the pull of gravity and to lighten your spirits. Strong standing poses with graceful stretching movements will make sure that you stay full of joyful energy and in great shape.

73 Ball of energy (2)

This is a repeat of Ball of Energy (35), which was introduced earlier in your pregnancy. It is included here to remind you that it is a wonderful workout that lifts your spirits, and is just as useful for this late stage. Keep your legs strong and your knees well bent to protect your lower back as you stretch and bend your upper body in all directions.

> **CAUTION**
> Do only what you feel comfortable and happy with, at your own pace and without strain. Take plenty of rest between sequences.

◁ **1** Take hold of your ball of energy in your hands. Take time to feel its weight and dimensions. Once you have its measure, start to play. Roll the ball between your hands, working your arms and shoulders.

◁ **2** Now roll your imaginary ball out to one side, twisting in your upper body as you do so.

◁ **3** Bounce your ball on the floor, bending forward and relaxing your neck. Remember to keep your legs strong but relaxed and knees bent.

◁ **4** Toss the ball in the air, opening your chest and arching your upper back. Continue to improvise in whatever way you like – the idea is to be creative and have fun, as well as exercise your body.

74 Dynamic hip opener and stretch

This is a fluid, dancing movement, expressing feelings of well-being and exuberance, lifting the spirits and opening the heart as well as lifting the upper body and opening the hips. It is excellent for creating lift in the upper body by stretching the arms up, which removes pressure around the diaphragm, and creating more space in the lower abdomen by opening up the hip joints.

△ **1** As you breathe in, raise one leg to the side with the knee well bent and the hip open. At the same time, stretch up your arms and lift your sternum.

△ **2** As you breathe out, gracefully lower your arms and bent leg. Then begin again with the other leg. Repeat these two movements rhythmically, so that they merge into one fluid dance movement.

△ Sometimes you may need a little help to make your yoga more fun. Enjoy these unscheduled moments.

"Delight in yourself, in the meditative movement and the dance you are creating...this yoga is truly a dance..."

Janine Parvati Baker

Stretches for a strong lower back and abdominal muscles

Think of yourself as an athlete in training who needs to build up power in specific groups of muscles for the task in hand, in this case giving birth. The muscles you will be using for childbirth are those in your lower back (for support and pushing against), your abdomen (to push the baby down the birth canal), your perineum and pelvic floor (for elasticity and control) and your breathing muscles (to make sure you stay energized throughout). You do not need complicated or expensive equipment in order to strengthen these particular muscle groups – you can find the props you need around your own home.

75 Kitchen yoga

Isometric exercises help to strengthen muscle groups and a good way to do this is to push or pull against an immovable object to create resistance. For these exercises, do make sure that what you are pushing and pulling against really is immovable.

◁ **2** Bring your feet in line as you stand facing a ledge or shelf. Get a good grip with your fingers and, as you breathe out, pull down hard, bending your knees and sinking into a half squat. Hang there, breathing deeply and stretching through your trunk and arms as you work the muscles in your legs.

◁ **3** Stand in front of a counter top with one leg forward and the other back. Lean forward, bending your knees, and place your forearms on the edge of the counter with your forehead on top. Now, push down to open your chest and upper trunk, taking the push through your back heel as you lengthen your lower back. Hold, then repeat with the other leg back.

△ **1** Stand in front of a wall unit (or a wall). Place one foot well in front of the other, with the front knee well bent. Lean forward and place your palms on the unit at head height. Adjust your position so that you are the right distance away to push hard. Breathe in deeply and push, taking the force down through your back leg. Involve all your abdominal muscles on the breath out as you maintain the push. Swap legs and repeat.

76 Stretch and squat with chair

Use a steady, upright chair to both stretch and squat down, as both positions will help to open up in the groin and stretch the pelvic floor. Keep your spine horizontal and your heels on the floor. To make the chair even steadier, push it against a wall.

◁ **1** Stand in front of the chair with feet apart and toes turning outward, so that your knees will bend over your feet at the same angle. Bend forward and hold the sides of the chair seat, keeping your back stretched and horizontal.

◁ **2** Squat down, bending your elbows to keep your back as flat as possible. Focus on stretching the inner thighs, the groin and the pelvic floor in preparation for giving birth. Breathe through this stretch, exhaling as you go down. Repeat frequently.

77 Perineal stretch with chair

Use a chair to help you when practising the Gentle Perineal Stretch (62) at this stage. For comfort, place a cushion under the shin and foot that you are going to sit on. This exercise will really help you to prepare your body for birthing. Finding the position in which your perineum is most relaxed and you can move your pelvic floor muscles easily is most important for this exercise – you might even get some kicks from your baby!

◁ Move from the Stretch and Squat with Chair (76) posture to a wide kneeling position, resting one knee on a cushion. Place the other foot out to the side of the chair. Now, holding on to the chair, press down and stretch through the whole perineal area on an out breath. Change legs and repeat the stretch. Practise frequently.

Relaxation throughout the day

Never miss an opportunity to relax, alone or in company. If you can relax the muscles that are carrying your baby at every opportunity, it will greatly enhance your feeling of fitness and well-being. Keep a beanbag handy for those blissful moments.

△ Kneel in front of a beanbag and flop over it to conduct weighty conversations with your toddler.

△ If someone can be gently massaging your thighs meanwhile, then so much the better. Relaxed enjoyment is the key.

Yoga movements for tone and energy

All these standing and walking movements help to create space in your abdomen and between your hips so that your baby has more opportunity to move around and get settled in a good position ready for the journey down the birth canal. So wriggle around as much as you can! In addition, shifting your weight from one leg to another, either in standing or walking poses, helps to prevent or ease varicose veins and swelling caused by an uneven distribution of your body weight.

78 Upper torso circles

These stretches lift your chest up and away from your abdomen, relieving pressure on your abdominal organs and giving your baby more room to change position. They help to diminish the effects of wind or gas in your digestive system and alleviate heartburn in the last few weeks of your pregnancy.

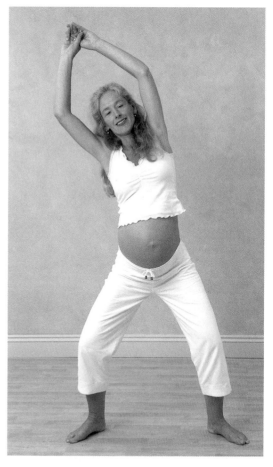

△ **1** Stand with feet wide and knees well bent. Stretch your arms overhead with hands clasped and palms facing the ceiling. Breathe in and stretch up some more.

△ **2** Make large clockwise circles with your clasped hands as though you were swinging a rope around above your head. After some clockwise circles, repeat the movements anti-clockwise. Engage the muscles at the sides of your body as you circle your upper torso and shoulders.

79 Pink panther strides

These exaggerated strides open the hips and pelvis, as well as the chest for deeper breathing. They work the muscles at the sides of the abdomen and spine. You will have to concentrate to make sure that you use the right combination of legs and arms at the right time.

◁ **1** Start off in a centred, firmly based standing pose with feet together. Now stride forward boldly with your left leg, swing your left arm forward and your right arm back. Freeze in this position.

▷**2** Making a big stride, bring your right foot forward along with your right arm, taking your left arm back. Holding in between, repeat these alternating strides. Now change to left leg forward, right arm forward and right leg forward, left arm forward, and repeat for a few strides. Then swap over again to left-left and so on.

80 Hip drops

This is another name for the famous "Charlie Chaplin walk". Hip Drops can be practised either standing on one spot or striding forward. This walk will ease pressure in your hips, pelvis and lower back and encourage your baby to join in and get moving. Try to get the rhythm of "strong then limp" in each hip as you wobble forward in an aimless sort of way with a silly grin on your face. This isn't as odd as it sounds – a tight jaw can be a sign of a tight pelvis. Your midwife may even ask you to drop your lower jaw during labour to relax your pelvis.

△ **1** Turn your feet out. Stand on your left foot. Drop your right hip, letting your right leg dangle loosely. Swing your limp right leg forward.

△ **2** Stand on your right foot with right leg strong, dropping your left hip and letting your left leg dangle loosely. Repeat.

Helping your baby move into position

You will find that your baby is sensitive to your moods, shares your enjoyment and joins in with all your activities. So the more that you dance around and stretch, and open and tone your body, the better he, she or they will like it. Your centre of gravity lies deep within your pelvis. The opening up of your hips and pelvic area, plus all the activity, will encourage your baby to find the very best position to be in as birth approaches. Putting aside time each day for a few minutes of energetic yoga dance, followed by perineal breathing, is the perfect way to prepare for labour with your baby. Don't forget that all these rotating, twisting and opening movements of the hips should be done with knees bent.

81 Knee circles

This is a balancing exercise that shakes out your hips and legs as you get into a knee-swinging stride. It is a loosening and strengthening movement, good for the circulation and for lifting your mood. If you feel wary about trusting your balance, place one hand against a wall for support. These knee circles should be done smoothly and lightly. Keep arms, shoulders and neck relaxed. The raised leg is also kept as loose as possible throughout.

▷ **1** Stand on your right leg, with arms spread to the sides at shoulder level for balance and your spine erect. Now swing your left knee up in front of you as high as is comfortable.

△ **2** Bring your left knee to the side to open your left hip and so make more room in the abdomen and pelvis.

△ **3** Now, swing it round behind you and kick back strongly with your left foot. Finally, swing your knee forward, straightening your left leg and placing your left foot firmly on the floor. Repeat with the right knee.

82 Pushing the sky

In this pose you are pushing your palms against nothing. The aim is to lift and strengthen your upper body and make space in your lower body as you flex your thigh muscles. It is an empowering position. Use your diaphragm and breathe deeply, involving all your abdominal muscles. This pose helps prevent or repair a split in the central band of abdominal muscles, particularly if you are expecting twins.

▷ **1** Stand with feet wide and toes pointing outward so that you can bend your knees deeply and hold this position. Keep your spine erect and raise your arms overhead. Now push upward even further with first one palm and then the other, turning your palm upward if you can and lengthening through each side of your body in turn.

◁ **2** Keep your arms directly overhead. Push upward while going into a semi-squat downward, lengthening through your middle on an out breath.

83 Standing twist

This is a good position either on its own, to ease tension in the neck and shoulders, or as a counter-pose to the strong sideways stretch of the Knee Circles (81). Breathe deeply and twist through the whole torso.

84 Seated perineal stretch

Now that your baby has grown so much, a low stool and several cushions are useful props for this modified version of the Gentle Perineal Stretch (62). Place one cushion on the stool and the others under your dropped knee as required. Remember throughout that it is the breathing that creates all of the action when you are stretching the yogic way – otherwise nothing happens, or you simply stretch a little in the groin area.

△ Place your right foot on a low stool or chair, with your thigh parallel to the floor. Raise your arms and open your elbows so your chest feels open. Place your palms behind your head with neck strong and straight. Breathe in. As you breathe out, twist your head and shoulders to the right. Your chest will follow, but your lower body is kept steady by the bent leg. Repeat the twist to the left, with your left foot on the stool.

△ **1** Sit on a cushion astride a low stool, with your knees wide and feet firmly planted on the floor in front. Stretch up through your spine by pressing your palms against your spread thighs.

△ **2** Pressing down firmly into your right foot, drop your left knee back and down on to the pile of waiting cushions, to stretch through the left groin and the perineum. Clasp your hands, breathing in as you push the palms away from you in a forward stretch, taking your weight through your strong right leg. Stretch further as you breathe out and lift through the spine as you breathe in several times. Change legs and repeat.

Preparing for labour with kneeling poses

Sitting on your heels, with a cushion between your buttocks and your heels for comfort, is one of the best positions you can adopt at this stage of pregnancy. Your spine is erect, with the coccyx hanging freely, and the trunk's weight is flowing down naturally through your legs and into the floor. This open position means that your baby's head has the maximum amount of space in your pelvis. With the padding from the cushions, you can comfortably maintain this position while you are doing other things, such as chatting to a friend. Kneeling poses also prepare you for a birthing position on all fours – a comfortable and popular choice.

85 Chest openers

Clasping your hands behind your back can be difficult for some people, yet it is well worth persevering because it is a good way to open the shoulders and chest, straighten the upper spine and make more space – especially to ensure a better position on all fours.

◁ **1** This is the classical position. One elbow is brought up to ear level and then bent to bring your palm against your upper back, while the other elbow is brought down by your side and bent to bring the back of your hand against your upper back. The two hands find each other (sometimes with help from a friend) and are clasped. They pull on each other to create the stretch at the front of the body.

△ **2** Take a few deep breaths in the position, then relax.

▷ Here is another chest opener with variations for different levels of suppleness in the shoulder joints. Take both arms behind you. For an easy version, hold each elbow with the opposite hands. For a stronger stretch, press your palms together behind your shoulder blades in the Namaste (prayer) position. Lean forward to stretch the spine at the back, making room between your knees for your baby. If leaning far forward is uncomfortable, then just lean a little way, or lean on to a low bed – whatever you are happy with.

86 Tiger stretch and relax (2)

Do you remember Tiger Stretch and Relax (1) (48)? It is important to carry on with this stretch in the final few weeks of your pregnancy, as it is an excellent way to revive the circulation in your legs as your growing baby presses upon the major arteries, veins and nerves in the lower back and groin. Alternate this exercise with the Active Kneeling Stretch (87) that is shown below.

▷ Begin in the Cat Pose (45). Stretch your right leg out behind you, parallel to the floor. Let it drop and trail out behind you, dropping your right hip. Shake it to relieve stiffness after kneeling or sitting. Readjust your position and do the same with the left leg.

87 Active kneeling stretch

Another good kneeling stretch for the final weeks of pregnancy. Alternate with the Tiger Stretch and Relax 2 (86).

△ **1** From a kneeling position, put your weight on both hands, lifting your upper body, and slide your right leg over to place your right foot firmly on the floor. Now raise your buttocks on an in breath and stretch your lower back as much as possible as you flex your bent right knee and open your right hip joint. Keep your weight equally distributed on your left knee, your right foot and your hands, using a gentle rocking movement. Repeat on the other side.

△ **2** This is a gentler version of the active kneeling stretch, using a bed, as you may not feel strong or supple enough to kneel on the floor comfortably as birth approaches or during labour. Kneel on a low bed, resting on your forearms, and let one leg drop toward the floor at the side of the bed. Breathe deeply, focusing awareness on your lower back. Repeat on the other side of the bed.

Massage, breathing and relaxation

These last few weeks are the time to take full advantage of all the help and support that family and friends can give you. You need to build up your reserves of physical and emotional strength in preparation for the birth, and the changes in your life once your baby is born. So rest and rest again, at odd moments and in whatever position you find comfortable. While relaxing, breathe deeply in order to nourish both your baby and yourself, and to let go of aches and tensions. Massage can be a great help, and the person doing it does not need to be an expert, as long as they are happy to do what you ask.

▷ Cuddles and closeness are especially soothing and sustaining during this final period of waiting. Let the whole family join in.

88 Back massage for deep breathing

This is one of the most soothing things that one friend (or partner) can do for another. It can be heaven for the recipient and also very soothing and relaxing for the person doing the massage. The recipient kneels with her knees wide and toes touching, and stretches over the beanbag in a relaxed and comfortable position. The beanbag will yield to fit the baby comfortably. The masseuse can kneel comfortably to one side, leaning forward slightly to massage her friend's back in soothing, circular movements. Both of you should make sure you are relaxed and comfortable before starting the massage. If pregnant herself, the masseuse should not lean forward too far, as this could cause backache.

◁ The masseuse lays both hands gently on the recipient's back and leaves them there for a moment. This establishes a gentle contact while she co-ordinates her breathing with that of the recipient. "Two breathing as one" is a key feature in massage. The masseuse then moves her hands as the recipient is breathing out (and therefore relaxing), lifting them slightly to allow the recipient room to breathe in deeply into her back lungs beneath the helper's hands. See exercise 49 for back massage guidelines.

89 Ankle massage in supported Warrior pose

The purpose of this exercise is to relax the thigh and calf muscles passively while a friend supports your stance and massages your lower leg. Leaning against a wall with your head on your hands lifts your upper torso and creates more space for you to breathe deeply into your abdominal, pelvic floor and buttock muscles. You will find that this brings blissful relief generally, and relieves tight calves and lower backache in particular. Cramping in the calf muscles is common in late pregnancy as your legs cope with the extra weight and your blood circulation slows down.

Preparing for birth through massage

Self-massage is a technique that pays great dividends in terms of ease during the birth and afterwards, as breastfeeding is being established. It is easy and relaxing to do, and well worth spending some time on. You do not need to use any oil for your massage, but if you wish to, then use pure plain oils as some oils are not recommended during pregnancy – check with an expert aromatherapist first. There are five main areas to focus on.

1 The base of the body, the perineum, has to be strong to support the contents of the abdomen, especially as your baby grows much heavier in later pregnancy. At the same time, however, it will also have to yield and stretch in order to let your baby pass down the birth canal. Nature provides for this change in texture by releasing "loosening" hormones that soften the ligaments. You can also help to improve elasticity in this area by self-massage. Massaging the yogic way can greatly increase the comfort and ease with which you give birth, and possibly prevent a tear or the need for a surgical cut (episiotomy).

2 Up to 36 weeks into your pregnancy, your breasts can be prepared for breast-feeding by regular massage. In Western societies, women's breasts are always covered up and so become unnaturally soft. Massage helps to tone and strengthen the breasts and make the surrounding areola more elastic.
3 The abdomen has to stretch a great deal during pregnancy and can be made much more elastic by regular massage. This also helps to prevent stretch marks.
4 Your feet and ankles may be swollen by fluid retention. Massage can often help to relieve this congestion, thus easing pressure and swelling and the resultant aches and pains.
5 While you have the massage oil on your hands, don't forget your face. Gentle circular movements over the face relieve tiredness and tension and feel soothing and relaxing.

how to massage yourself

You may like to take a relaxing bath first or just apply a hot, wet flannel to the area to be massaged. The hot flannel brings the blood

△ **Massaging the muscles around your mouth is helpful for keeping your lower jaw dropped and your face generally relaxed during labour.**

closer to the surface, which is soothing in itself. Settle yourself with the oil, if using, beside you. Find a comfortable, supported position. Reclining is probably best, either against a beanbag or on your bed.

Apply a little oil, if used, to your hands. Your touch should be exploratory but relaxed and gentle, indeed almost passive and reflective. Use your breathing actively as part of the massage. The stretching of tight skin and tissues is not caused by your fingers but by the relaxation of the tissues against your fingers when you breathe out. So, whatever part you are massaging, work with awareness of your breathing, moving your fingers on the out breath.

▷ **Massage your breasts with gentle strokes, going toward the areolas. Do not massage the nipple area itself (see the Caution box) and avoid any breast massage after about 36 weeks.**

> **CAUTION**
> **Nipple massage**: Do not massage the nipples themselves. However, if you have reached your due date, then tweaking your nipples gently between thumbs and index fingers can be an effective way of stimulating producton of the hormone oxytocin and so helping to bring on labour.
> **Perineal and vaginal massage**: Never pull or attempt to stretch these tissues manually.

"From early days,
Beginning not long after that first time
In which, a Babe, by intercourse of touch
I held mute dialogues with my Mother's heart..."

William Wordsworth

◁ **Very gentle abdominal massage helps to prevent stretch marks.**

perineal massage

It is truly amazing just how quickly the normally tight tissues in the perineum, vagina and abdomen will stretch with regular massage. The more that you are able to pre-stretch these tissues before the birth the better you will return to your original shape after it. Start around 36 weeks and practise once a day.

Use a light touch to explore the layers of tissues along the back wall of your vagina and the skin that separates your vagina and anus. It is this area that will be most stretched during the birth of your baby and is most prone to tearing.

Insert two fingers into the vagina up to the first knuckle, progressing to the second knuckle with practice. Press against the back wall of the vagina, against the spine, while breathing deeply. Feel the muscles under your fingers as they engage on the breath out. As space is created, move in further and exert a little more pressure. Using your breath in this way is like blowing up a balloon. Nothing much seems to happen at first, but soon your perineal tissue starts to give and then begins to stretch. You will be amazed how much you can stretch it, simply by breathing out into the areas under your fingers.

▷ **Massaging swollen ankles and feet relaxes the tissues here, which allows your blood and lymphatic fluids to circulate more freely, bringing nutrients to the area and removing waste products and excess fluid.**

▽ **Most women find that the most comfortable and convenient position for massaging the perineum and vaginal areas is reclining on their side against a beanbag or bed.**

Yoga for labour and birthing

Day by day, your baby is getting ready to be born. Your body responds to your baby's signals with practice contractions of your womb and the release of birth hormones. This is a time of great excitement and some uncertainty, of exhilaration and suspense. You need yoga more than ever, to create and maintain feelings of peace and surrender in preparation for your baby's journey into the world. All your stretching and breathing practices will come into play during labour and the birth itself.

the labour circuit

Each birth is unique and each labour starts differently. As you approach your due date, it can be helpful to choose and practise several positions to use during early labour. These should keep you comfortable and help you to breathe through your contractions, making them as effective as possible. These positions make up your "labour circuit". The labour circuit allows you to stay in your own unique rhythm and to ease the descent of your baby by making full use of gravity. If all goes well, it may help you right up to the point where you are fully dilated. Every 15–20 minutes, move from one position to another position around your circuit. You will find that one or two positions will begin to feel the most comfortable and secure and you will tend to stick with those.

From time to time, also use movements 79 (Pink Panther Strides) and 80 (Hip Drops). These will loosen up your hips and back and release tension. Alternating positions is particularly helpful if labour is slow to get established, as this helps the baby's head to press down on to the cervix. What follows are some suggested positions for inclusion in your own labour circuit.

> **CAUTION**
> Make sure the surfaces you lean against during your labour circuit can support your weight.

91 Supported squat against the wall

These positions help engage the muscles of the abdomen and the lower back to assist uterine contractions during labour. They also make full use of gravity to open the cervix effectively as well as to alleviate pain, particularly in the lower back. To conserve your energy, lean against the wall with your elbows resting on a windowsill, and a stool in position in case you need to sit down.

▷ **1** Stand with your legs a comfortable width apart. Now adjust your position until your back is supported by the wall as you bend your knees in a semi-squat position.

◁ **2** If this position puts too much strain on your thighs and legs, or you already need to sit down to breathe through regular contractions, lower yourself down the wall until you are sitting on the stool, still with your legs apart. Make sure that your back is upright against the wall.

92 Standing poses during labour

After squatting for a while, stand up and practise the Pink Panther Strides (79) and Hip Drops (80). When you feel a contraction starting, try these supported standing poses as they are an effective way of facilitating the descent of your baby's head. You may prefer to press down on a chest of drawers or counter with your hands rather than against the wall, but in the same standing position. Circling your hips rhythmically can feel very soothing.

◁ 1 Face a wall and lean against it. Bend your knees and press against the wall with your forearms, resting your head on top of your joined hands.

◁ 2 Then, keeping your forearms in the same place, bend your knees and let your hips drop down on an out breath. "Hang" in this position and breathe deeply, focusing on the out breaths.

93 Supported kneeling

Supported kneeling is a favourite labour position for many women and can provide you with periods of active rest during your labour. It can also be a good birthing position. It is important to adjust the position of your knees so that they are not too wide apart for comfort. Take time to install yourself in such a way that your spine is extended as much as possible while the shoulders remain relaxed. Cushions or pillows can be placed under your knees and feet for greater comfort if you need them. This position is especially soothing if you experience backache during labour, particularly if your baby is lying in a posterior position – that is, with his or her back to your back. Change position again after 15–20 minutes.

▷ 1 Use a beanbag or exercise ball to stretch your back during labour. A ball is excellent as you can move back and forth slightly, which is highly soothing. Hug the ball and rest your head on your arms to keep your neck comfortable.

◁ 2 Use a windowsill or high bed if you prefer a more upright position. Support yourself with your forearms and make sure your neck and shoulders are relaxed.

△ 3 Kneeling over a low bed with your arms above your head gives your shoulders a particularly good stretch.

Yoga breathing for labour

Many of the complications of labour arise from physical exhaustion, often made worse by lack of sleep, so you need plenty of deep rest as the birth approaches. Conserving your energy is also a priority from the moment you discover that labour is starting, and the best way to achieve this is through deep breathing that follows the rhythm of your contractions. Taking a sip of water after each contraction is helpful too. When you are fully dilated, the breath takes on another role by helping you to give birth with minimal strain.

breathe out to welcome the contractions, then let them go

In the first stage of labour, most women have contractions at intervals that gradually become shorter as the labour progresses. From the very beginning, your most important task is to relax as much as possible between the contractions and to avoid dissipating your energy, particularly by talking. Your breath out needs to be used for getting rid of tension as the contractions come and go. During each contraction, focus on breathing as deeply as you can, depending on its strength. Then start to relax again, even if only for a minute.

◁ Kneeling on all fours, keeping your head relaxed, can be a very effective position for grounding you and helping you to cope with backache during labour.

centring with breath during labour

Your labour circuit positions may involve your partner, who can be holding you or massaging you, or you may prefer to labour on your own, drawing deeply upon your inner resources. Whichever way is best for you, the ebb and flow of your breath can help you to remain centred through awareness of the flow of breath – both during and between your contractions. You will find that breathing is your most powerful tool for surfing the contractions rather than attempting to resist them. After any conversations or medical procedures, use your breath to re-centre yourself.

◁ Each time you feel a contraction on its way, breathe out deeply. This allows you to welcome it with relaxed muscles, and this, in turn, helps the contraction to work more effectively to open your cervix. Breathe throughout the contraction in whatever way feels best for you. When the contraction peaks, it is time to breathe out again deeply, to send it on its way and to dispel as quickly as possible the inevitable tension that results from pain.

▷ Sitting astride a gym ball allows you to use gentle pelvic rocking, in time with your breath, to relax between contractions and to centre yourself once more.

breathing for birthing

The second stage of labour begins when your midwife confirms that the birth passage is fully open and ready for your baby to pass through. You may already be feeling a strong urge to push your baby out, or you may feel nothing at all. Every woman is different. The two priorities in all cases, however, are to relax as deeply as possible to make space for the baby, and to relax all the muscles of the pelvis, particularly those in the buttocks, for birthing.

When it comes to breathing, voicing your breath out, on any note that feels good to you at the time, helps the abdominal muscles to work together with the powerful bearing down contractions. The longer that you can extend the breath out, the farther your baby is able to move down the birth passage during one contraction. Engage your inner pelvic muscles on your out breath, pushing from within. Try to keep your facial muscles, and the rest of your body, as relaxed as possible as you do this, to lessen the strain.

Your midwife will guide you as to when, or if, you should breathe lightly – as if you were blowing on hot soup. This need arises if you have to hold back and wait for your perineum to stretch as the baby's head crowns. By blowing lightly, you are disengaging your abdominal muscles from your breathing and so weakening the impact of the uterine contractions.

◁ Voice your breath out with a "Haaa!" sound deep into your lower abdomen. Extend it for as long as you can to increase the pressure of your contracting uterus on your baby's body as he or she moves down the birth canal.

Gravity, centring and a voiced breath out can be combined in a powerful yet light action to push your baby out. Let awareness of your baby guide your breathing. Breathing your baby out into the world is a loving action that is open to most women and brings many possible long-term benefits to both mothers and babies. Even if medical intervention is necessary during your labour, breathing and relaxing with yoga will facilitate any birth process.

breathing to deliver the placenta

To deliver the placenta after the baby is born, use the same breathing that you employed for the birthing.

Zoë's story

Mine was a highly positive birthing experience – due to my husband's very vocal encouragement and essential breathing advice from Françoise. Having attended a yoga class throughout my pregnancy, I felt well-prepared, but when contractions suddenly started on my due date, I was taken by surprise by the strong back discomfort. I stayed at home for as long as possible with my husband and friend, timing contractions and pushing on my back to relieve the pain.

When I arrived at the hospital, my friend and husband arranged my pillows, sat me on my birthing ball and set up my specially chosen music. I started to meditate, breathing through the contractions. After a long labour, where the contractions hit me hard, and I became rather frustrated by watching the head bob back and forth for a couple of hours, I heard the word "episiotomy" from my midwife and with one contraction focused on my breathing and pushed five times to deliver my wonderful daughter, Kira.

Yoga and birth positions with a partner

For many thousands of years, women in all cultures have given birth in positions that make use of gravity, although for much of the last century, Western hospitals tended to encourage women to give birth on their backs. The advantages of not lying flat on your back for giving birth have now been recognized and currently women are encouraged to sit up, or to lie on their side, for delivery on hospital beds. This is a step forward, although here we present further birthing positions that allow you to be more active still. If you have practised yoga regularly during your pregnancy, these positions should feel both familiar and comfortable. Supported standing in a semi-squat, supported squatting and variations on kneeling are all possible options that you can try out beforehand to discover which one feels best for you. Some women consistently favour a leaning-forward position while others prefer to lean back. Supported birth positions also mean that partners can be actively helpful and closely associated with the birth of their baby. In this book we refer to a male partner, but of course you can enlist the help of a female friend.

94 Birthing: supported standing positions with partner

The supporting partner must be confident that his back is strong. He leans against a wall with his feet a little away from the base of the wall and his knees slightly bent to ensure a strong bracing position. Stand as close as possible to your partner. You must feel able to let go completely, trusting that your partner's back is pressing against the wall and that he can take your weight safely during contractions. Both of you should relax between contractions.

△ **First position** Face your partner and link your arms around his neck. Bend your knees and let yourself hang down.

△ **Second position** Stand with your back to your partner. Let him support you with his forearms under your arms while you bend your knees in a semi-squat.

95 Birthing: supported squatting positions with partner

Women who feel that they can create more space in their pelvis when they are leaning back can experiment with this position in one of its variations. The first variation is an extension of the standing semi-squat, which can also be used with a birthing stool.

△ **First variation** 1 Use the support of a low stool so that you can squat easily while hanging from your partner's shoulders.

△ 2 During the final birthing contractions, touching your baby's crown can help you to pace and centre your breathing.

△ **Second variation** Your partner sits behind you on a sofa while you sit on the edge, between his knees. Holding hands helps you both to centre your breathing in close harmony with each other.

△ **Third variation** Your partner sits on a chair legs apart and back straight, supporting you under your arms as you drop into a wide squat. Adjust your feet so you are as straight and relaxed as possible.

96 Birthing: supported kneeling positions with partner

If you choose to spend a major part of your labour on all fours, then a supported kneeling position may be the best birthing option. There are many variations, depending on how you choose to kneel, the angle of your back and the height at which your partner sits to support you. Be guided by your experience as you focus awareness on your pelvic floor. Put cushions under the knees for comfort.

△ **1** Kneel in front of your partner, putting your arms around his neck for support. This position makes good use of gravity and relieves pain if the baby is pressing against your lower back.

△ **2** Kneel as before, but this time spread the knees wider and sit further down. The tilt of your pelvis can be modified to widen the birth passage. Let your body guide you into the best position.

△ **3** Kneel as before, then bring one foot forward outside the knee. This position allows the widest opening in a position that may combine the advantages of both squatting and kneeling.

new
mothers

After the joy of welcoming your baby
into the world, you may remember
the firmer, slimmer body of early
pregnancy and wonder if, when and
how you will wear those clothes
again. Trust the power of the breath in
toning the deepest muscles in your
body. They are your best allies to
developing not only a fine figure but
also your future strength.

Basic breathing techniques

Before you start any postnatal exercise, the first thing to focus on is your breathing. We call this "Yoga Breath Awareness". Watch yourself breathing. Become aware of your breath just as it is. Then, without forcing your inhalation, very gently extend your exhalation, allowing your natural breath to become gradually slower and deeper. This can have a profoundly calming and settling effect at any time. The breath is closely linked to the nervous system. Shallow breathing will make you physically tense, mentally distracted and emotionally anxious. Deep breathing has the opposite effect, making you centred and steady.

A deep breath in will quite naturally charge body and mind with new energy, and a deep breath out will release muscular tension, chemical waste products and feelings of tiredness and strain. For this reason, you should breathe deeply and slowly at all times during yoga practice, and the book will also give you guidance on when to breathe in or out. This joining of mind and body through breath and movement is yoga. After a few days' practice, you will be able to use your breath in many new ways.

You can use Alternate Nostril Breathing to energize and/or calm yourself, and Reverse Breathing to tone the deep muscle layers of your abdomen and spine. Take every opportunity to practise and perfect these breathing techniques. A good time to do this is while you are feeding your baby, as long as you can remain relaxed while you are practising.

1 Reverse breathing

During pregnancy you may have used breathing exercises to open the body, make more room for the growing baby and facilitate the birthing process. Now the situation is reversed: your aim is to close the lower part of your body, pull the stretched muscles inwards and upwards, and strengthen them so that they hold the spine, pelvis and abdominal organs in correct alignment. This is the purpose of Reverse Breathing. Practise for a few rounds, or until you feel tired or lose your rhythm. Stop and rest, and repeat whenever you feel ready. With practice, you will feel very toned and strengthened after breathing in this way.

△ **1** Sit or lie comfortably, with your spine supported. Place your hands on your lower abdomen, to become aware of what is happening. Breathe in deeply, imagining the energy of the breath being drawn up through the base of your body into the abdomen.

△ **2** As you breathe out, pull in your waist, drawing your navel up and closer to your spine at the back. Feel this out-breath continue to flow up into your chest, toning you powerfully from inside. Release at the end of your exhalation. The out-breath is longer than the in-breath, but this shouldn't be forced. You can take a "resting breath" in and out before inhaling and drawing up again, or repeat the Reverse Breathing without a pause.

2 Alternate nostril breathing

This exercise works on the nervous system, quickly soothing the emotions and calming the mind. Use it whenever you feel stressed, as well as part of your daily routine. Two complete breaths form one round: do several rounds. Your breathing will deepen naturally – never force it.

△ **1** Sit comfortably and erect. Bring your right hand in front of your face, with the three middle fingers tucked in towards your palm and the thumb and little finger extended. Place your thumb on your right nostril to close it, and breathe in through your left nostril.

△ **2** Close the left nostril with your little finger and breathe out through the right nostril. Holding the hand position, breathe in through the right nostril, then close it with your thumb, open the left nostril by lifting your little finger and breathe out through it.

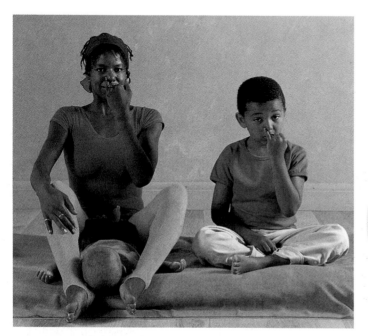

◁ **Whenever you feel the need for energizing, perhaps just after your baby has gone to sleep, a few rounds of Alternate Nostril Breathing will refresh you in two to three minutes. You can invite other children to do it with you before you play with them too.**

"The moment I first touched my new born, a love I had never felt before swept my heart."

Feeding and energy

You will enjoy your new baby most if you are feeling good in yourself. This good feeling largely depends upon two things: regaining your fitness and vitality, and being able to rest and relax despite the inevitable lack of sleep. Fitness and relaxation are the two keys to happy mothering and a happy baby, so these are the two "arms" of yoga that we will be focusing on in this book. Everyone in your family will enjoy the benefits of your yoga practice.

No sooner have you welcomed your baby into the world than feeding becomes an all-absorbing task. However well prepared you have been for this, it takes a great deal of adjustment for both your baby and yourself. Relaxing in a comfortable position can make a significant difference to your early experience of breastfeeding and make it more enjoyable from the start. If you are bottle-feeding, practising "yoga breath awareness" can contribute towards creating a closer physical bond with your baby.

feeding positions

In the first weeks following birth, it is important that your back should always be well supported when you breastfeed. You may prefer a reclining position at first, in bed or on a sofa, but favour an upright position as soon as this is comfortable. If you

△ While sitting up or reclined, make sure your lower back is well supported. Use a cushion to raise the baby's body if needed.

had a Caesarian section or a traumatic birth experience, lying down with your baby at your side may continue to be your most

◁ If you had a Caesarean section you will need, at first, to find positions where the weight of your baby does not rest on your abdomen.

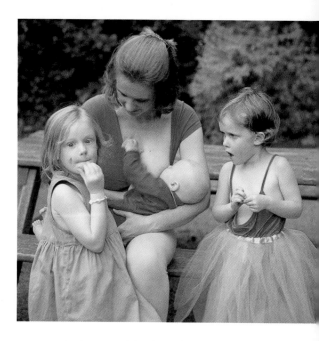

◁ As you grow stronger you will be able to feed your baby in a variety of positions. The important aspect is relaxed comfort.

▷ If you were in the middle of doing something else when the baby wakes for a feed, take a few deep breaths before you pick up your baby. This allows you to transmit a message of loving nurture to your baby, rather than one of irritation at being interrupted.

comfortable feeding position for longer. If needed, raise your baby on a cushion so that your back can remain straight while you feed. If you are sitting on a chair, you may need to place a cushion or use a support to raise your feet so that your knees and hips are level. Check your feeding position again and again, week by week, anywhere you happen to be with your baby, to make sure your back has adequate support while you feed. You spend so much time in feeding that forming good habits with regard to feeding positions is a fundamental step in regaining, or creating, a sound posture after birth. Always relax your shoulders.

breathing and relaxing while feeding

Feeding your baby is a precious time to practise breath awareness and save, if not generate, energy. Once you are settled in a comfortable position, use a deep exhalation to release any tension you hold in your body at the time. If you are breastfeeding, you can do this while the baby is "latching on" and

while hormonal changes are occurring in your body. Slow down your breath, using the "yoga breath awareness" technique, and feel that you are beginning to rest. If your baby does not feed easily and gets frustrated, start again calmly. Early obstacles can be overcome more easily and rapidly if you can break for relaxation while feeding your baby. Then feeding becomes a positive rest time in which you can practise some other breathing techniques, such as "reverse breathing", and also relax deeply while

remaining close with your baby. Making the best use of feeding times to renew and save your energy as a new mother is one of the main aspects of regaining fitness and vitality the yoga way.

bottle-feeding

It is even more important when bottle-feeding to breathe yourself into a welcoming, nurturing attitude before you pick up your baby. Relax while the baby is awake and alert at the beginning of the feed.

▷ Hold the bottle at a comfortable angle for your baby to suck on it. Relax and enjoy this moment of physical closeness and rest with your baby.

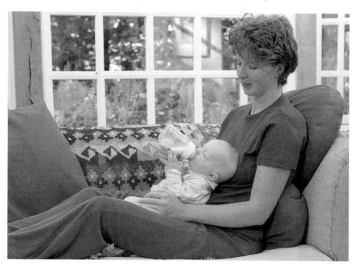

The art of relaxation

new mothers

Yoga relaxation involves four elements: slow, calm breathing, comfortable posture, physical and mental relaxation. Slowing your breathing right down and breathing out slowly will calm the nervous system. You may already know, or will soon discover, how rapidly and well this works through your practice of expanded breathing. Relaxation is both a tool and a completion.

basic relaxation

In relaxation you do more than rest. You enter another state of being in which you are neither sleeping, nor engaged in activity. Think of it as putting your gearbox in the neutral position, disengaging from all your voluntary thinking and acting.

The more you stretch all the muscles of your body with yoga, the easier it becomes to relax them. The more you breathe in your stretches, the deeper your breathing becomes and the more you can make use of your breathing to either energize or quieten yourself. Life with a baby changes from day to day, nearly from moment to moment. Before you learn the classic yoga relaxation in Shavasana (27), or Corpse Pose, it helps to practise this basic relaxation whenever you can, through the day and night.

Although you will relax more deeply if you can lie down, any position in which you can settle comfortably for a minute or two is

△ Lie on your back with your head, neck and spine in a straight line. Avoid letting your chin poke upwards by lengthening the back of your neck. Let your arms lie stretched out loosely, a little away from your body, with the palms up and fingers gently curled. The shoulders and upper back are spread wide and soft. Stretch out your legs, with your feet apart and rolling slightly outwards.

△ If you intend to relax deeply for ten minutes or more you may wish to cover yourself with a shawl (and socks in winter), as your body temperature will drop. Include your baby and relax deeply together.

◁ If your pelvis tilts in this position, making a hollow under your waist, you may be more comfortable bending your knees and placing the soles of your feet flat on the floor to begin with, until in time your back remains flat with your legs outstretched. Meanwhile, press your back gently towards the floor as you breathe out.

▷ Once you have learnt how to make your body "let go" on demand, you can practise relaxation in many positions and situations. This is the Child Pose (67) which we look at later in the book.

fine. Inhale, then extend the exhalation as much as you can. If you feel that you need to, then voice it, or Haaah, or yawn it, a few times. Then close your eyes and be aware of your breathing. If you have learnt to breathe in your abdomen while pregnant, feel yourself breathing deeply. Then let go of your conscious breathing and feel yourself resting. Experience the quality of rest that results from relaxing in stillness and quietening your breathing. At this stage you are entering the open space of relaxation, where your whole physiology can be refreshed and restored.

mental relaxation: use the power of visualization

This aspect of yoga practice helps you to let go even more, releasing tensions within your body and also within your mind. Imagine yourself in a happy scene, such as lying in a beautiful garden. Build up this scene and make it very real for you. Bring your baby into your visualization. Feel close and bonded, with both of you basking in the sunshine of universal love, both

▷ Once you have learned the art of non-doing you can slip into this mode of being anywhere, any time you wish.

▽ Learning to relax and let go creates space for quality time with those we love.

of you being nurtured together. Include others who are close to you in this happy scene. Feel loving and loved... After a while, let the vision fade away, knowing that it is always there for you to recapture. Focus on your breathing and start to come out of your relaxation.

emotional relaxation: the attitude of surrender

This is the true purpose of your relaxation: to let go, to surrender to the flow of life, to be rather than to do. Learning to "go with the flow" makes a mother's life happier and her relationships more rewarding.

You can relax deeply while you are feeding your baby – to the great benefit of both of you. Use relaxation to help you to go back to sleep during disturbed nights, or to soothe your baby to sleep.

Breath, relaxation – and now movement

By increasing your awareness of your every-day movements, you can eliminate a great deal of postnatal tiredness and strain. Consciously allow your legs and upper back to carry your weight – and often that of your baby as well – rather than relying on your lower back and abdominal muscles. If you had a Caesarean section or episiotomy you will need to be especially vigilant while the scar tissue is healing. Practise the following exercises regularly, to restore muscle tone in the perineal and abdominal muscles. When these muscles are weak, the spine and pelvis move out of alignment, causing both poor posture and lower backache.

3 Reverse breathing II: for the pelvic floor

Practise the first stage of Reverse Breathing for a while, until you feel absolutely comfort-able with it. Then add the following: as you breathe in, tighten and pull up the perineal muscles at the base of your body, drawing them up into the abdomen. Tighten the muscles at the centre of your "seat" (the vaginal muscles), drawing also on the back (anal muscles) and the front area (the muscles that hold your bladder in). This exercise, when practised regularly, can save years of discomfort and problems – including stress incontinence and prolapse – caused by perineal muscles that have been overstretched during childbirth.

Continue to tighten these muscles even more as you breathe, releasing them at the end of your out-breath. Practise using these sets of muscles in a smooth, wavelike flow of the breath. This exercise can be done almost anywhere and at any time. Rest for a few seconds between breaths, or between sets of six breaths. To alleviate any problems due to the weakness of your perineal muscles, do two sets of six breaths three times a day for two or three weeks.

4 Getting down to the floor and up off the floor

Getting down to the floor and up off the floor is something new mothers soon find themselves doing many times a day. If you have done yoga during pregnancy, you will already be familiar with the "all fours" position, called the "Cat Pose" (25). If not, why not start enjoying the benefits of this pose right away to soothe your back and avoid straining it as you go down to floor level and up again. This first basic sequence introduces yoga movement in your life as a new mother in a simple but effective manner. In yoga, body symmetry, suppleness and stretching are constantly practised so as to eventually become effortless during everyday activities.

▷ 1 Once on the floor, position yourself on your hands and knees in a firm, symmetrical and well-balanced position "on all fours".

▷ **2** To get up off the floor, lean forward first so that you can easily turn your toes under. Then, in one flowing movement, walk your hands on the floor towards you while rolling your back to find yourself sitting on your heels, as shown. Remember to keep your neck relaxed.

△ **3** By stretching your legs and pushing on your hands you find yourself getting up off the floor in one easy movement. With your legs bent at first, then extended, you can now stretch your spine to a full upright posture. Your lower back has been protected at all times during this sequence.

△ **4** Practise going down to the floor again on all fours by bending your knees and extending your arms towards the floor, palms stretched out. Your heels will probably lift from the floor as your knees reach down. Stretch on all fours and get up off the floor again, making this a rolling motion up and down.

Your first yoga routine

Every woman progresses at her individual rate, depending upon many factors: how well she is after the birth, how dedicated she is to her yoga practice, how busy her life is, and how well the baby is settling down. Some days flow smoothly whilst others seem to snarl up. The most important thing is to do what you can – today. Yoga is totally non-judgmental, so to compare yesterday with today is pointless. Every day is an opportunity to progress towards greater pelvic strength, better alignment of the spine, deeper relaxation, more serenity and inner balance. The weeks after giving birth bring huge changes, physically, emotionally and mentally. Your aim is to relax and heal, to energize and tone your body, your emotions and your mind. Regular deep breathing will keep you on course even when your emotions are all over the place. Above all, make time for rest.

If you have just a few minutes to spare, remember that relaxation comes before stretching. Alternate Nostril Breathing (2) is instantly relaxing – you will stretch all the better afterwards. If you are interrupted, take a few deep slow breaths to give your practice a completion.

yoga in the first six weeks

The routines here include postures on the floor (lying down, sitting and kneeling) and a few standing postures. Exercises can be practised on their own, or one page or more at a time.

Make sure that you do not do too much, too soon. The exercises included in this section are designed for the first six weeks after giving birth. You can continue, with great benefit, to do them for the rest of your life. But please do not go beyond them, to the next stage, until six weeks have passed. Even then, please wait if you do not feel ready for new challenges. It is far better to practise simple routines regularly, and to grow stronger and more relaxed, than to push yourself too fast and become stressed.

5 Legs up the wall

Even if the birth was relatively easy and you feel fit and well, take time to practise your Reverse Breathing (1) with your legs raised. If your birth was difficult, or you had a Caesarian section, it is important to tone your inner muscles with deep breathing. In the position below, the floor and wall will give you a solid support to help you to expand your abdominal breathing.

△ **1** Sit sideways against the wall. The aim is to place your legs parallel against the wall.

△ **2** Bend the knee nearest to the wall, leaning back on your hands.

△ **3** Swivel round on your bottom, leaning back now on your forearms. Straighten your legs and move your upper body round.

▷ **4** You should be lying in a straight line with your legs together, hands on your abdomen. Flex your toes, lifting your heels, to strengthen your legs.

△ **5** You can strengthen your abdominal muscles by bending one knee and placing the sole of your foot on the wall, then repeating with the other leg. Remember that, after giving birth, you are working to close your body, so keep your legs together to tone your inner thigh muscles more effectively.

△ **6** Once settled in this position, you can include your baby. He or she will enjoy closeness with you, lying peacefully against your heart. Without even moving, you are using the calm power of your deep breathing to tone the lower back and abdominal muscles.

abdominal and lower back muscles

After your baby is born, lying flat on your back again is a new feeling. It is also the first, the safest and the best way to re-align your spine and tone the pelvic muscles in depth after giving birth. Feel your lower back settle into the floor and open up. One or both knees stay bent at all times to protect your lower back and ensure that you remain relaxed while you stretch. As your uterus returns to its normal size, yoga breathing allows toning through all the layers of abdominal muscles.

6 Knees to chest

In this exercise, Reverse Breathing (1) is used to tone the muscles of the lower back, together with the pelvic floor. Vaginal tone is also improved. If you have had a Caesarian section, do the first part – no. 1, below – only, for several weeks.

△ **1** Lie on your back with your knees bent and your feet flat on the floor. Stay comfortable and relaxed. Breathe freely in your abdomen.

△ **2** Clasp your hands below your knees and, using Reverse Breathing (1), breathe in, drawing your pelvic floor muscles up, then further up as you exhale.

◁ **3** Inhale again and pull your thighs closer towards the chest as you breathe out, bringing your waist down towards the floor and widening your upper back. Repeat a few times.

7 Leg over

This exercise introduces a gentle twist which helps tone your transverse abdominal muscles as you practise your yoga breathing.

▷ Straighten one leg along the floor and place your other foot outside it, bending your knee. Place both hands on your abdomen. Breathe deeply, drawing your abdominal muscles in towards your spine as you exhale, and pressing your feet on the floor.

new mothers

upper back and shoulder muscles

The exercises on this page aim to tone the dorsal muscles that were supporting your baby inside you, in your "bump". It may seem both enjoyable and strange to feel and regain ownership of this space with your yoga breathing. If your baby is awake you welcome him or her into your practice. Yes, baby, here you are, out in the world, but still close to your mother.

8 Hug yourself

This exercise helps to open your upper back and at the same time to recover the sense of your body as your own after giving birth.

◁ Fold your arms across your chest, with fingertips on opposite shoulders. Hug yourself and breathe deeply, feeling the expansion in the back. As you exhale, press the base of your spine on the floor and let your whole back spread out.

9 Side stretch

This stretch elongates your spinal muscles. As you breathe more and more deeply between your hips and your ribcage, feel your waistline again.

▷ Straighten one leg along the floor. Bring the arm on the same side over your head and stretch it along the floor behind you. The whole of this side of your body should feel stretched and open. As you breathe in, flex your foot and stretch your arm, extending from heel to fingertips. Stretch more as you breathe out. Release and relax. Repeat several times, then change sides and repeat with the other side. You can also stretch diagonally, extending opposite arm and leg one way and then the other. Breathe the same way.

10 Namaste

The pressure of the hands held together in this Indian greeting allows you to breathe more deeply in your upper and middle back. At the same time, you build up inner strength in your open heart area.

◁ Lying down with your knees bent, join your palms together in front of your heart, in the prayer position. Inhale and press on your palms as you breathe out slowly. Feel the upper back and shoulder muscles strengthening and the front of the chest lifting. At the end of the practice, relax.

Regaining strength and stamina

As you practise the stretches that follow, use Reverse Breathing (1), which will help you stay relaxed and to stretch further. If any area feels tight or tense, breathe out into it to relax it before continuing. Start your stretch from the lower back or pelvis – that is where strength enters, with the breath in. Keep your body relaxed so that you experience the flow of breath while you are stretching.

11 For leg and abdominal muscles

Lie on the floor, reclining against a beanbag or other support. Make sure that your lower back is well supported and your shoulders and neck can stay relaxed. This is a flowing movement in which your legs alternately extend and bend with a relaxed stretch, toning the whole abdomen. If you are able to stretch your legs completely without tensing your abdominal muscles at this stage, you can do so.

◁ **1** Inhale as you extend your relaxed leg up.

△ **2** Then bend your knee.

△ **3** Exhale slowly as you extend your leg towards the floor. Extend your leg up again as you inhale and enjoy a smooth circle of movement and breath.

12 For abdominal and pelvic floor muscles, lying down

Practise this exercise as often as you can. Lie on the floor with your legs propped up on a bean-bag or other support.

▷ Bend one knee towards your chest and clasp both hands around your shin. As you breathe out, press your knee to your chest while you also pull your navel up and back towards your spine. This makes your chest widen at the back and lift at the front. Release the pull on your leg before you breathe in again. Repeat a few times, then change leg.

13 For abdominal and pelvic floor muscles, sitting

Sit on a cushion on a firm chair. If you have a Caesarean scar, place a large, soft cushion on your lap to protect your abdomen. Keep your back very straight and your waist against the chair back.

△ Pull your knee to your chest, pressing your foot on the chair. Use Reverse Breathing (1) pulling your knee towards the chest on the breath out. Repeat several times on each side. Keep your face soft and your neck relaxed.

14 For upper back muscles, lying down

Lie on the floor with your legs on a beanbag or a pile of cushions for similar support. Make sure your lower back is comfortable on the floor; if it is not, raise it with a pillow. Relax both your lower back and your legs.

◁ **1** Raise one arm as you breathe in. Stretch it up and then behind your head as you breathe out slowly. Flop the arm back to your side at the end of your out-breath.

◁ **2** Repeat with your other arm. After a few rounds, work with both arms together. Make sure you keep the back of your waist in contact with the floor throughout, even if you cannot reach the floor behind you with your arms.

15 Wall stretch

Many new mothers find that the weight of their enlarged breasts makes their upper back droop and ache. If you feel like this, the "wall stretch" will help you extend your spine and use deep abdominal breathing to tone and open your back muscles. This stretch also helps prevent mastitis as the overall circulation in the breasts is improved.

△ **1** With your knees hip-width apart, kneel on a cushion in front of a wall so that when your hands are flat on the wall, your spine is straight.

△ **2** Keeping your tailbone tucked in, let your hands slide down the wall very slowly while you breathe as deeply as possible.

△ **3** Feel your whole spine stretch as you sit on your heels. Continue to elongate your spine for a few breaths. Repeat for a few rounds, or rest.

Spinal stretch

After extending your spine on the floor in the lying down exercises, sitting postures practised on a chair enable you to stretch further and strengthen your lower back from the base of the spine. Sitting upright will also help you to practise Reverse Breathing (1) and pelvic floor lifts more intensely against gravity, as you are working.

16 "Sun wheel" stretch

Sit on an upright chair with your spine erect and feet planted firmly on the floor. Pull your spine upwards from its base to the crown of your head. Keep your neck long and your shoulders down and relaxed.

▷ **1** Breathe in. With your out-breath, push your palms down towards the floor, fingers facing out to the sides and wrists bent back in line with your spine. Your shoulder blades draw closer together and your chest expands. Push as if you were moving air currents away from you on the out-breath.

△ **2** Bend your elbows and raise your hands higher as you breathe in, then repeat the downward movement, pushing more on the out-breath.

△ **3** Next time you breathe out, push your palms out to your sides at chest level. Keep a flowing movement, breathing in and out.

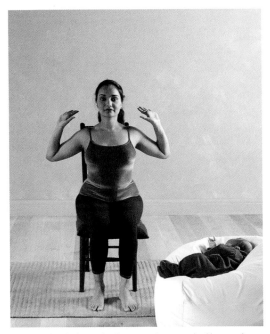

△ **4** As you breathe in your hands are now above your shoulders, opening your upper back and stretching your chest and arm muscles.

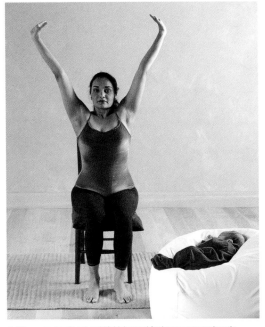

△ **5** Turn your hands out and lift higher and further on your out breath, opening the rib cage. Enjoy your full span, stretching to your fingertips.

△ **6** On the next round, lift your arms straight up above your head, stretching more as you breathe in. Start your downward wheel by reversing the steps, breathing in your own rhythm with a slow movement.

△ **7** When you have completed your "sun wheel", bring your hands together into a seated Namaste position. Press the palms together and breathe quietly, enjoying the effects of this sequence on your whole back.

Gentle twists and bends sitting on a chair

Twisting movements are central to yoga. They are powerful toners, firming the body from inside out in the abdomen and around the waist. Practised gently to begin with after giving birth, twists and their counterparts, forward bends, are very effective means to help new mothers "close" their body again after opening it to grow their babies and give birth.

Yoga twists start from the base of the spine, involving the lumbar area and then progressively the whole back. They stimulate the functioning of all the organs, as the leverage helps you breathe more intensely in the abdomen and chest together. It is usual to twist to the right first, then to the left, as this sequence follows the line of flow in the large intestine. In sitting twists, make

sure you keep the spine stretched up as you twist, from the lower back to the shoulders. The head follows rather than leads this upward slow movement which you expand with your breathing. Twisting is always done on the out breath, and with each out breath, you twist a little further. Today's limit will seem easy after only a week's practice, but never force, just let the extension come.

17 Simple twist on chair

The first twist can be practised soon after giving birth to regain your awareness of your waist. It also opens the chest which helps when you start feeding.

△ **1** Allow your right arm to hang down loosely by your side. Place the back of your left hand against the outside of your right thigh. This hand is your lever: press it against your thigh to help you to twist to the right. As you breathe out, start the twist at the base of the spine and continue it all the way up, so that your neck and face turn last, and you are looking over your right shoulder. Release the twist a little as you breathe in, then increase it as you breathe out again. You can make this simple twist stronger by holding the back of your chair with your right hand. You now have two levers to help you, pushing away from your left hand and pulling towards your right hand. Come back slowly, to face front, as you breathe in.

△ **2** When you have finished, bend your right knee and pull your shin towards your chest as you breathe out. Then twist and bend to the left side. Repeat all these twisting movements to the left.

18 Circling one arm

This is a gentle stretching twist that counters the tension of feeding and stretches the spine. Do it often.

19 Crossing your legs

This twist allows a long diagonal stretch that is invigorating.

△ **1** Sit upright on your chair, with the back of your left hand outside your right thigh. Stretch out your right arm behind you.

△ **2** Breathing deeply, make a slow circling movement with the extended arm. Repeat on the other side. Then, use your right hand as the lever as you twist to the left and circle your left arm.

△ Cross your left leg over your right knee and – if you can – tuck your toes behind your right calf. Use your left hand as the lever, pressing it against the outside of your right thigh. Twist to the right, circling your right arm in a wide sweep up in front and down behind you, breathing deeply. Repeat on the other side.

20 Forward bend (1)

Bending forward after giving birth may feel slightly uncomfortable at first. You have not been able to bend for a long time, and now bending may remind you that your body has changed. Trust that yoga will help you tone your body in depth day by day. If you have had a Caesarian section, place a pillow on your lap before bending forward.

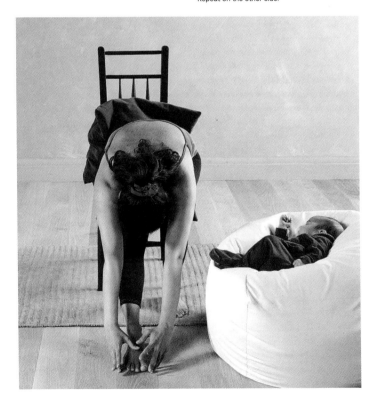

▷ When you have finished the twisting movements, relax completely. Extend your right foot along the floor and ease your lower back by flopping forward, breathing out. Extend your arms to your shins, ankles or, if you can, to your toes. Repeat with the left foot, and then extend both feet, breathing deeply with long, slow, relaxing breaths out.

Basic kneeling sequence

These movements strengthen and relax the whole body. They will give you a good workout, improving flexibility and lifting your spirits. The movements should be learnt separately, then practised as a routine that flows with the rhythm of your natural breathing. If you have done yoga before, you may recognize a kneeling version of the "sun salute". In this version, you remain close to the floor to avoid straining your abdominal muscles, which are not yet ready for the full sequence. The exercises are also complete in themselves and can be practised separately. Always relax at the end of the kneeling sun salute. You can return to the Swan Pose and rest or lie in Shavasana (27). Try to get into the habit of relaxing, even for a minute, after completing every sequence.

24 Swan pose

In this relaxing pose, the stretched arms help you breathe more deeply in the middle and lower back. This can be very soothing.

▷ **1** Relax and stretch in this pose, sitting on your heels. Extend your fingers forward for maximum stretch. Press on your hands when you exhale.

◁ **2** Bending your right arm so that your forearm can rest on the floor, stretch your left arm forward as far as you can, extending your fingers. At the same time, allow your spine to extend backwards, breathing into the stretch which reaches from your hand to the base of the spine. Change sides and repeat.

▷ **3** Bend your elbow to open your chest fully. Rotate the shoulder, breathing into the circular movement of your bent arm. Replace your forearm on the floor and work the other side. Change sides and repeat. Rest afterwards with your head and arms down, as before, if you feel tired.

25 Cat pose

This is an easy way to stretch your spine. In a steady "on all fours" position, alternate an upward and downward circling of the back together with an inhalation and an exhalation.

△ **1** Go on all fours, with your back flat. Your knees should be hip-width apart: the hip directly over the knee and the shoulder over the wrist. Spread your fingers for good support. Breathing in, arch your spine and tuck your head in.

△ **2** Breathing out, flatten your back at the waist and look up. Repeat. If you wish, you can create a flowing movement, bending your arms to roll back and forth in the stretch.

26 Leg stretches

Lower backache is common in the weeks after giving birth. Leg stretches can both prevent and ease tension, particularly around the sciatic nerve.

△ **1** Starting in the Cat Pose, above, breathe in and bring one bent knee forward towards your face, keeping the calf muscle and foot relaxed.

△ **2** Breathing out, stretch that leg out behind you (keeping it relaxed). Your body, from crown to heel, stretches in a straight line. Extend your out-breath as much as possible.

◁ **3** Turn your extended foot inwards and drop it on the floor, relaxing your leg and trailing it limply, allowing the hip to drop. From this position, bring your bent knee forward again to repeat the three steps several times. Then change legs.

Healing relaxation from six weeks

This relaxation is not just to recover from your exertions after a yoga session or to rest after a disturbed night. It is for healing, and for integrating the whole experience of pregnancy and childbirth into your life.

The period of six weeks after giving birth is known as "postpartum". The six-week point signals the ending of one phase and the start of another, as you cease to be a "new" mother and become instead a mother. As you pass from one stage to the next it is important to avoid taking any unnecessary physical or emotional baggage with you. You want to move on feeling healed and whole, ready to enjoy your baby.

Six weeks is about the average time it takes to recover from giving birth. For you it may be shorter or longer – you will know when you have reached this dividing line. But even when the birth experience is many months behind you it is still a good idea to do this focused relaxation from time to time. It helps you to assess how well you are moving on into the flow of your life, and free remaining areas of tension.

conscious surrender

This pose seems very simple, but it involves considerable body awareness, which only comes with practice. Breathe the tension

"As I sit quietly with you my child, I ask that I be made a strong and loving parent. May your life always be filled with light."

away, then move on to visualizing your happy scene in which you are experiencing total well-being.

From that contented space, look at any unhappy feelings that sometimes afflict you. Be brave and honest with yourself. Acknowledge your own feelings of tiredness and low spirits. Accept them as part of how your life is, and how you are.

We are all just as we are. Judgment and perfectionist standards (your own or anyone else's) have no place here. Simply soothe and care for yourself, just as you would for a dear friend who came to you for loving support. Be your own dearest and most reliable

friend – and learn to accept help from this source of inner strength.

You may become aware of other feelings, too. Unacknowledged anger is common: anger at the disruption to your life since your baby was born, anger at feeling disorganized, anger at other people, anger at having to put aside your own interests. These are just a few of the issues that may come up. You may also experience feelings of sadness: grief for the time before you had responsibilities, or for

▽ **As you quieten the body and the mind in stillness, allow this conscious relaxation to free you from fluctuating emotions.**

the loss of your own childhood, or for those golden days when you never seemed to run out of energy.

Mixed emotions are normal at this stage, around six weeks after the birth. They may come as the result of changes in lifestyle, or hormonal changes as your body returns to its pre-pregnant state, or a mixture of both. The first step in dealing with any such feelings is to admit that you feel them. Then tell your "inner friend" all about your sad or angry feelings and ask for understanding, support and healing. These are already there

for you – you have only to ask. Emotional burdens can be lifted from you simply by acknowledging them and sharing them with that "inner friend" who loves you and whom you know you can trust. Be humble and true to yourself as you do this.

Having accepted and then released your negative feelings, you can fully experience and share all your feelings of love and joy. Take time to allow them to surface. Tell your baby of your great love, and tell the other members of your family that you love them, too. Draw them all together into the circle

of your love. Recognize and be grateful for the deep joy that is welling up within you and radiating outwards to everyone around you. Breathe gently in and out of your heart space for a few moments.

When you are ready, let the vision fade away. Become aware of your breathing and expand it slowly until you are back in focus. Then move your fingers and toes. Finally, s-t-r-e-t-c-h and yawn before starting to sit up. Remember that the deeper your state of relaxation, the more important it is to come out of it slowly.

27 Shavasana

Refer back to the basic relaxation technique, although by now it should be second nature to you. Your position should be a comfortable one that you can maintain without moving. Shavasana, or the Corpse Pose, is a classic yoga relaxation pose. Once you are settled and comfortable, avoid any further movements. Close your eyes and just let go. Scan your body from the inside and, wherever you find any tension, melt it away and nurture that space. Do the same with any images or emotions that arise, connected with your birthing experience.

To come out of the pose, expand your breath gently but steadily, until you feel drawn to open your eyes effortlessly. Feel your body come back into focus. Then stretch before you sit up. Relaxation is progressive – each time you practise, it helps you to go deeper next time.

◁ Lie down comfortably, at a time when you can expect to be undisturbed for at least ten minutes – hopefully longer.

◁ If it is more comfortable, you can have your head and shoulders supported by a beanbag or pillow. Relaxation can be practised in bed when you need it.

Pulling up

Realigning the spine after giving birth may take time and dedication. But persevere because it is a very important process which lays the foundation for your future well-being as it may determine your long term posture. "Standing tall" refers not only to having a straight back, but also to using your pelvic floor, abdominal muscles and lower back muscles to hold your pelvis in perfect alignment with your spine. Then stretching becomes truly beneficial... You will look and feel amazing.

28 Tadasana: standing tall

This is a classic yoga pose and is used as a starting position for many others. With a vertical support, use your awareness in this pose to realign the spine after pregnancy. You can line yourself up against a wall or the edge of a door, to get into the correct position, and then take a step away without losing your "line". Reverse Breathing (1) will greatly assist you.

◁ 3 After breathing in position 2 for a while, straighten your legs again and stand tall against the door. Check your best position today. Breathe deeply, feeling your alignment. Every day will be different.

◁ 4 After doing this you can also practise standing on one leg and circling the other foot inwards and outward, exercising your ankles and feet arches.

△ 1 With your knees loosely bent and your feet a foot's length away from the door or wall, line up your spine all along its length. Pull up the lower abdominal muscles as you breathe in. Bring the waist back and open the chest as you breathe out. Draw your chin and neck back.

△ 2 Bring your heels close to the door. With your hands, explore the hollow behind your waist. Bend your knees slightly, more if you have done yoga before, to align your spine. Remove your hands. Use Reverse Breathing (1), to strengthen your back muscles, drawing in your pelvic floor muscles – deep as you inhale and further as you exhale.

Protecting your lower back

Babies soon get heavy and it is easy to strain yourself when lifting and carrying them around, particularly in seats and carriers.

Remember that your abdominal muscles are likely to be overstretched from giving birth, so they cannot do their normal job of

protecting your lower back. Compensate for any weakness by making the best use of your leg muscles and upper back.

29 Standing up, holding your baby

Your baby may join you on the floor while you practise your yoga, change a nappy, or breastfeed between sequences. Several times a day, practise getting up from the floor, and getting down, holding your baby with your back strong and straight. You will soon develop strength and poise.

△ **1** Kneel, then rise to one knee, using your arms and upper back to support the baby's weight.

△ **2** Take your weight on to your front leg, turning the toes of your back foot under, and rise.

△ **3** Straighten your knees only after your spine is erect and you feel balanced.

30 Bathing your baby

It is common for new mothers to strain their backs while bathing their babies. Yoga helps you to develop an awareness of the way in which you reach forward and can lift your baby most easily.

△ **1** Kneel on one knee, as close to the bath as possible, with a towel at the ready.

△ **2** Take a deep in-breath as you lift your baby, completing the lift on an out-breath.

△ **3** Sit upright as you dry the baby.

Yoga every day

Once the basic techniques in this section have become really familiar to you, any spare time can be used for yoga. Here are some suggestions, and you will soon discover other ideas yourself. Be creative! Remember to use Reverse Breathing (1), and to practise your deep relaxation daily. Always rest for a few moments after yoga breathing and stretching.

yoga breathing
Get into the habit of using Reverse Breathing (1) at any time of the day or night, whatever position you happen to be in. Every breath in draws the energy of life – of vitality and healing – into the abdominal cavity to strengthen and tone the stretched muscles of the perineum and abdomen.

Every long breath out allows the energy of love – of openness and relationship – to lift the chest and the spirits and to open the upper back and the heart space. As these two aspects of universal energy blend, and flow up the spine to the crown of the head, you feel a light energy in and around you. Your mind becomes focused, clear and serene and your posture upright and confident.

The benefits seem purely physical at first but, as you continue to practise, you will find that deep and beneficial changes occur; you are being healed at many levels. This is the magic of yoga.

relaxation
This is an essential part of any yoga session. Always include a resting position after every

sequence and a relaxation at the end of your session. Rest is healing and deep relaxation will replace lost sleep. Alternate Nostril Breathing (2) is a quick and effective way to centre yourself at any time, and a good way to begin each yoga session.

good posture
Use Reverse Breathing (1) to help draw yourself upright every time you feel that you are drooping. Use your upper back and leg muscles to take the strain off your abdominal and lower back muscles.

stretches
Always start your stretches from the lower back. Avoid tensing your legs or arms – stay loose and use your breath to extend further.

31 Minding your posture in the kitchen
While you are waiting for the kettle to boil, or for something to finish cooking, you can realign your posture and practise Reverse Breathing (1) to tone your abdominal muscles in depth from the pelvic floor.

△ **1** Strengthen your thigh muscles by bending your knees. Support yourself by bending your elbows behind you and leaning on a table or chair back.

△ **2** Bend and straighten your knees, keeping your spine erect and your chest open. As you stand up, inhale and lift, exhaling as you bend.

◁ You can lean against a wall in any spare moment, drawing up your spine and keeping it in contact with the wall.

▷ Remember your posture when doing housework. Aim to keep your knees bent and your spine erect. Bend your knees before leaning forward or lifting anything.

△ Stand in front of a long mirror from time to time to check your progress.

△ Stop, relax and enjoy life whenever you can – it is time well spent, time that will not return. Babies grow very quickly and the days rush by.

gentle
progression

Rest, more rest and relaxation come before

exercise. Each yoga posture becomes a

therapy in itself that stimulates but also

calms you, energizes but also nurtures you

in a comfortable, effortless way. Take time

to watch your body rhythms and your

feelings as you stretch more without ever

straining, letting your breathing guide you.

Six to twelve weeks after birth

The next set of exercises is more demanding, and should provide just what you need from six weeks to twelve weeks after giving birth. You will have had your postnatal check-up and are now probably ready to move on to some more classic yoga.

Everyone is different, however, and you should check your progress before moving on. You may have practised less than you would have liked over the last six weeks. You may feel that you still need to stick with the earlier routines for a while longer, for any number of reasons.

One reason may be that you have only just acquired this book! If this is the case, it is essential first to familiarize yourself very thoroughly with the basics of Reverse Breathing (1), relaxation and stretching.

The yoga techniques in this chapter form the foundation for ongoing physical, emotional and mental well-being. One of the ancient yoga texts emphasizes that, "In yoga no effort, however small, is ever wasted." However advanced you may become in your yoga practice, you should still make time to stretch and relax daily, and to be always conscious of your breathing and your posture. It takes only a minute to

"Nothing prepared me for the highs and the lows, the challenges, the defeats and the victories. It took weeks to become a mother and still be who I am."

practise a few reverse breaths, pulling yourself up from the perineum to the crown and opening your chest and your heart space. Get into the habit of doing this several times every day, wherever you happen to be.

The routines in this section will help you to consolidate your pelvic strength and the realignment of your spine. Some more yoga "asanas" (poses) will be introduced, as well as vigorous limbering sequences that really get the energy flowing. You will continue to breathe deeply and to make relaxation your priority – this is an essential ingredient

within every movement as well as during your rest afterwards.

Sometimes you may have only a few moments to spare. If your baby needs your attention when you are in the middle of a routine, go back to your starting position and take a deep breath out to relax. Then smile, as you go to greet your baby.

▽ **As you get ready for more active yoga, remember that relaxation is the foundation for renewing your strength and stamina from within. Keep using the relaxations from the first section.**

More advanced reverse breathing

The following positions – described in order of difficulty – allow you to get a really good "grip" on your pelvic floor muscles as you breathe in and out. You are now using the buttock muscles too. After pregnancy, it may be unfamiliar to you. First become aware of the power of your buttock muscles, tightening them and then releasing them, before practising the exercises on this page.

32 Standing against the wall
Tightening your buttock muscles intensifies the "pulling up" that you practised in Tadasana (28).

◁ **1** Stand with your heels a short distance away from a wall. Place your spine against the wall, knees bent. Tightening your buttocks, breathe in and pull the pelvic floor up. Hold the grip as you breathe out, then relax all the muscles. Repeat several times.

◁ **2** For a more extreme posture, raise your arms against the wall as you breathe in and repeat the exercise several times.

33 Raising the hips
Tightening your buttock muscles as well as practising Reverse Breathing (1) makes this apparently easy raising of the hips from the floor a very powerful toner.

△ **1** Lie on the floor with knees bent and feet flat on the floor, hip-width apart. Lengthen the back of your neck and keep your chin tucked in throughout. Place your arms alongside your body, palms down, to support you.

△ **2** As you breathe in, lift your pelvis up from the floor as high as you comfortably can, keeping your inner knees in a straight line. Grip the base of your spine with your buttock muscles and hold as you breathe out. Lift your pelvic floor again as you breathe in again, then relax as you breathe out.

△ **3** On your next in-breath, release the buttock muscles and lower your pelvis slowly to the floor, lengthening your spine as far towards your heels as possible. Repeat several times.

34 Lying prone
This position is one that you won't have been able to achieve for some time whilst pregnant. Now, it offers you a different angle for pelvic floor lifts.

△ Lie on your front with cushions under your breasts and your upper back wide and relaxed, with your elbows bent at eye level and your face turned to one side. Let your feet roll apart. Grip the base of your spine with your buttock muscles. Breathe in and out a few times, then release.

Standing sequence: stretches and balance

In this chapter, like the last, the yoga poses have been modified to provide you with a gentle progression, and are especially useful for those new to yoga. If you find any of these poses too difficult for now, do not worry, you can simply compose a sequence to suit you from the other poses in this section. Many standing poses can also be practised more easily with your back against a wall. If you stand a half-foot away from the wall, you can then use it as a support for your back by leaning against it while in the pose.

Some standing poses are described here as rhythmical sequences. Movement that flows with the breath is relaxing, effective and more "yogic" than a stretch in which you try and conform to a pre-set notion of how you should look in a posture. Before you feel comfortable holding "asanas", the word for classical yoga poses which implies steadiness of body, breath and mind, you can practise at least some of them using movement and rhythm. When you hold a pose, however, the dynamic is created inside your body with breathing. This is what makes yoga poses enjoyable. Whenever you feel tension, come out of it and relax.

35 Dynamic archer pose

As you become stronger day by day, stand tall in Tadasana (28), which is also known as the Mountain Pose, and feel the strong vertical axis between earth and sky.

▷ **1** Stand in Tadasana (28). This is the starting pose for standing postures in yoga.

▷ **2** Jump or walk your feet about 1m/3ft apart. Turn your right foot out, your left foot in. Inhale, raising your arms open to shoulder level without tensing. Exhale, bending your right knee and turning your head right, extending both arms. Inhale, straighten your legs, centre your head and turn left foot out, right foot in. Exhale, stretching to the left. Continue alternating sides.

36 "Easy" triangle pose (Trikonasana)

Find an easy rhythm, stretching only as far as you can go without disturbing your relaxed breathing. This sequence combines a stretch (the Archer Pose) (35) and an open twist in the Triangle Pose.

◁ **1** Begin in the Archer Pose, above. With your feet still apart and your arms extended, tilt your trunk to the right. Breathe naturally, letting your right hand slide down your right leg to the point where you feel you cannot go any further down without bending forward. Lift the inner arch of your right foot.

▷ **2** Keeping your weight on the left leg, inhale and stretch from your left heel all the way to the fingertips of your left hand. Look at your left hand and stretch more as you exhale. Come back to centre and repeat on the left side.

37 "Easy" forward bend

It is pleasant to let gravity stretch your spine while your shoulders, neck and head can relax completely in this forward bend, which also stretches the back of your legs.

▷ When you have stretched both sides a couple of times, come back to the centre and lower your arms to flop into a gentle forward bend. Relax your neck. You may like to swing your head and shoulders gently from side to side, to ease your lower back. Bend your knees as you breathe in to come up from this pose.

38 "Easy" tree pose (Vrkasana)

Start with a low chair or stool for this pose and graduate to a higher one as you become more confident and flexible. (You may prefer to have your back against a wall to do both this pose, and the Eagle Pose (Garudasana) (39), if your balance is unsteady.)

△ **1** Stand in Tadasana (28), facing the chair. Place one foot on the chair and bring your hands into Namaste (10) (the prayer position). Use deep breathing to stretch and align your spine and centre your energies. Hold the pose with your body, breath and mind remaining steady.

△ **2** Bring your knee up towards your chest, with both hands clasped below your knee. Keep steady and balanced, with your spine in line. As you breathe out squeeze your bent leg towards your body and release as you breathe in. Breathing deeply, hold the position for a moment. Release, regain your balance and steadiness, then bend the other knee and repeat.

Kneeling sequence: stretches, bends and twists

Sitting on your knees enables you to lift your lower spine and stretch without straining your lower back and abdominal muscles. Yoga "asanas" in this position straighten your back and make your spine strong and supple. They also tone your thigh muscles in a way that may surprise you at first. They remove fatigue and refresh your whole body with little effort.

43 Vajrasana

This is a classic sitting pose in which you can develop the awareness of your vertical axis – from the pelvic floor to the crown.

◁ Sit on your heels with your feet stretched out flat behind you and your spine and head erect. You may place a cushion between your buttocks and your heels if this is more comfortable. Use Reverse Breathing (1) to pull up your perineum, bring your waist back, open your chest and "sit tall".

44 Kneel tall

In this dynamic version of Vajrasana, left, the flow of breath assists the lift of the diaphragm in a rhythmical stretch up and down.

◁ Bring your hands together in front of you. As you breathe in, raise your buttocks, keeping your spine vertical and tailbone tucked under, and lift your arms above your head. Breathe out as you sit back. Breathe in and rise again and, if you can, hold for a few breaths before sitting back.

45 Chest expansion

This exercise is both a stretch and a forward bend. The challenge is to find the position in which your arms can stretch the most while your chest can open the widest. Make sure your neck remains relaxed throughout.

△ **1** Clasp your hands behind your back, sitting tall. Bring your arms up behind you, keeping them as straight as possible and squeezing your shoulder blades together.

△ **2** Next time you breathe out fold forward from the hips, keeping your arms raised. Breathe in, sitting tall. On the out-breath, fold forward from the hips and lift your clasped hands, opening your chest as wide as possible. Keep expanding forward, breathing as deeply as possible.

△ **3** Aim to place your head on the floor (or cushion) in front of you, still sitting on your heels. Breathe deeply and work to bring your arms higher with each breath out. Release your hands and come up on an in-breath, sitting in Vajrasana and observing the effects of the exercise.

46 Kneeling twist

Twisting in Vajrasana is slightly more difficult than the sitting twists on a chair presented earlier (17–19). Make sure you can kneel comfortably, with a straight spine, before you practise this kneeling twist. It allows further rotation and therefore is stimulating and enjoyable, even more so when you add a circling movement of the shoulder.

▷ **1** Place the back of one hand against the outside of the opposite knee and the other hand on the floor behind you. These are your levers. Sit up very straight as you breathe in and turn as you breathe out. Improve your twist with successive breaths out. Keep your neck relaxed and only turn your head to the extent that your spine twists. Eventually, you find yourself looking backwards without strain.

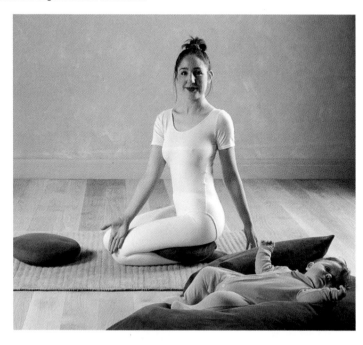

◁ **2** When you are ready, bend your back elbow and put your fingertips on your shoulder. Circle your elbow, loosening your shoulder and upper back. Repeat on the other side.

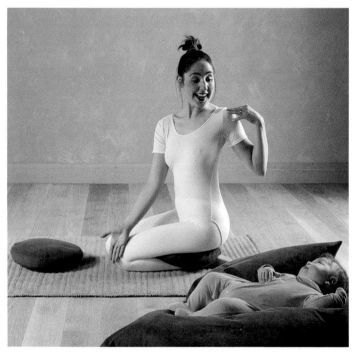

"Look at today for it is life.

The very life of life."

Kneeling roll

This sequence offers an expanded version of the Cat Pose (25). It is a stepping stone between the full "kneeling sun salute" (24–26) which keeps you grounded in your practice, and the classic sun salute of all yoga schools. We are giving a great deal of attention to this sequence because if it is not done correctly you may weaken your lumbar area when you move on to the full sun salute. Make sure you use your breath fully in time with the rhythm of this exercise, which is known as the "kneeling wheel".

47 Rhythmic kneeling sequence

Repeat this rhythmic, rolling movement several times to loosen and relax your whole spine. The sequence is based on the Cat Pose (25), kneeling on all fours. Check that your knees are directly under your hips, hip-width apart, and that your hands are under your shoulder joints.

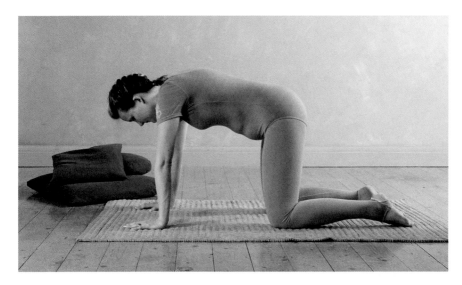

◁ **1** Begin with your back flat, with your neck and spine in a straight line. If you wish, practise the Cat Pose (25) first, stretching and arching your spine alternately on the in- and out-breath.

◁ **2** Lean back as you breathe out, opening up the lower back. Keep your arms fully extended (your hands have not moved at all) and lower your head as you stretch back. Ideally, your head comes to touch the floor while you remain seated on your heels.

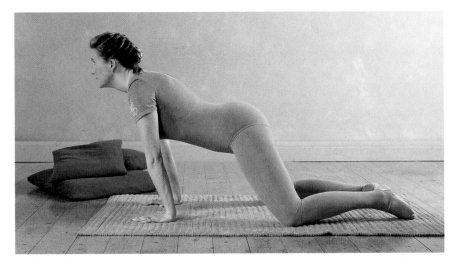

◁ **3** Inhale, extending forward on your knees and bent arms until you have to straighten your arms and raise your head to come up, moving your weight on your hands and lifting your shoulders.

◁ **4** As soon as you reach the limit of both your in-breath and your stretch, start rolling your shoulders to extend backwards with your arms straight on a long out-breath.

◁ **5** At the end of your out-breath, you are ready to bring your elbows to the floor again and start stretching forward on a new in-breath, extending your back fully again, as above. Keep your head relaxed. Enjoy the "wheel" movement with the flow of the breath in and out. Then relax.

From kneeling to sitting

gentle progression

From kneeling in Vajrasana (43), on your heels (or on a cushion placed on your heels) you can now move on to Virasana, a pose in which you sit between your heels (or on a cushion between your heels). This pose tones your abdominal muscles further and allows you to make Reverse Breathing (1) even more effective. You can use it as a base to stretch backwards and up. Virasana makes sitting straight in Dandasana easier as well as preparing you for the forward bends of classic yoga with a fully extended back.

48 Virasana

For this classical yoga kneeling pose you sit between your feet. If you find this pose difficult, place rolled cushions between your thighs and sit on these – it will get easier with practice.

▷ From a kneeling position, adjust yourself to make a comfortable descent towards a cushion or the floor, supporting yourself with your hands as you lower your buttocks between your feet. Make sure you can sit straight. Practise Reverse Breathing (1) in this position.

49 Back arch

Virasana allows you a full expansion of the chest and a stretch of the spine by moving your hands back in an easy back arch.

△ Breathe in and, as you breathe out, take your hands back with the fingers pointing forwards. Lower your weight on to your palms and breathe in deeply to open the chest and arch the spine. Take several deep breaths. Come out of it as you went in, crawling your fingers back towards your buttocks.

50 Push away

An upward stretch in Virasana knits your right abdominal muscles back together after pregnancy. If these muscles have split, practise this pose frequently for repair.

△ Bend your elbows and push your palms away from you, following the seated sequence described in detail in the Sun Wheel Stretch (16). This exercise is very effective to tone your right abdominal muscles. Exhale slowly on the way up, breathing in before you start pushing again from below.

51 Dandasana

This is a classical yoga sitting position. The word means "pose of a stick". You can use it to stretch your spine and legs before you relax after completing a sequence of kneeling poses. Put on some more clothes, so that you don't get cold, and place a beanbag, or a big pile of cushions, in position.

◁ **1** Sit close to the beanbag. Stretch your legs out, with your feet flexed. Place your hands near your buttocks and use them to push your spine upright and at a right angle to your straight legs. Use Reverse Breathing (1) to help you lengthen your lower back. Feel how you are sitting up taller and taller as you breathe. Your leg muscles are also toning as you lift yourself more from your buttock bones on the floor.

▷ **2** Raise your arms on an in breath and push away with your palms as you exhale, keeping your head relaxed. Bend your arms again as you inhale and push them further up as you exhale. This is a graceful but very demanding rhythmical stretch in which nearly every muscle in your body gets involved! If you find sitting on the floor too difficult for now, sit on a cushion or on the edge of a beanbag.

▽ **3** When you feel really stretched lie back on the beanbag and totally let go... perhaps alone, perhaps with company.

Making yoga part of your life

The breathing, movements and relaxation that make up your yoga practice will extend naturally into your everyday life. Take a few moments at frequent intervals to check the pattern of your breathing, the sense of "energy flow" in your movements and the state of relaxed contentment in your heart and mind. Make yoga a part of your life with a few appropriate exercises, wherever you happen to be.

At this stage your life is becoming more outward-looking, as you begin to resume your normal interests outside the home and you may be preparing to go back to work. You need flexible daily routines that suit your baby, your family and yourself.

Caring for yourself is still important. Maintain a special place in your own home where you can turn inward in deep relaxation to address concerns and feelings that are very personal. Your "yoga corner" can become the projection of your inner space, as you and your baby transform week by week.

When you nurture yourself during deep relaxation, you also strengthen the bond with your baby and dissolve stress around you. Yoga practice can become the tool for your transformation into a well-adapted mother. Whether you are at home or at work, you can refresh yourself daily.

52 Carrying

When you are sitting on a chair with your baby on your lap you can practise "pelvic rolls" to ease out your lower back and gain flexibility and awareness in this area. Use them to help you get up from the chair, and practise the same movements in reverse every time you sit down. They can also be used to get in and out of cars.

◁ **1** Arch your lower back, then tuck your tailbone under. Repeat this in a rolling action.

◁ **2** When you stand up while carrying your baby, tuck your tailbone under and bend your knees while keeping your back straight.

▷ **3** Let your thighs carry your weight, while your arms and upper back carry your baby.

53 Easy lifting

Use this technique for heavy shopping, but remember that babies in seats also constitute heavy loads, and they get heavier as they grow. So you will feel much more comfortable if you apply the principles of yoga from the start.

△ **1** To loosen up, bend your knees then straighten your legs as you stretch one arm, or both arms. Bend again as you release your arm or arms, and continue swinging in a rhythm; inhale as you stretch, exhale as you release.

△ **2** Pick up your load at the beginning of the upswing movement, as you inhale. Before lifting, your legs are bent and your arm is relaxed.

△ **3** When lifting a heavy load, always use both hands. Again, make sure that you are on the upswing, with your legs bent and your arms relaxed, beginning your inhalation. Feel your abdominal muscles are involved, but do not strain.

▷ **4** Lift as you inhale, keeping your knees bent and your back straight. You may find this makes greater use of your arm muscles, but your back is protected. Put a heavy load down in the same way, but in reverse order, breathing out as you let go of it. Relax your lower back and abdomen as you exhale (all the way down).

Yoga up and down stairs

Unless you live in a bungalow, you will find yourself going upstairs and downstairs many times a day with your baby. You may also have to carry piles of linen and clothes, and Moses basket, carry cot or baby seat. This sequence will help you to protect your back and also to stretch your spine as you go up and down. Make the stairs a prop to regain or gain fitness each day, with yoga.

54 Stairs

Going up and down the stairs, bending and extending your legs while keeping your back straight can make a striking difference to your energy level at the end of the day.

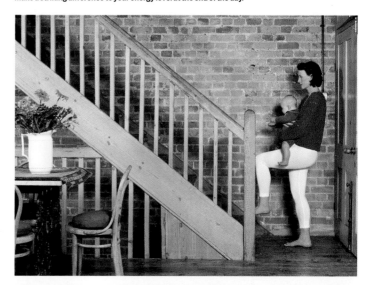

▷ **1** Going up, lift your bent knee really high and stretch up before you take your weight on your top foot. With practice, you can learn to inhale as you bend and exhale as you stretch.

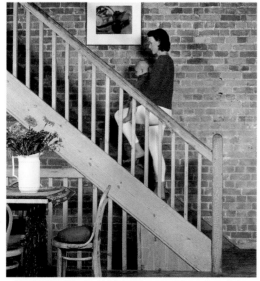

△ **2** Practise shifting your weight from your stretched back leg to your front bent leg, extending your leg muscles fully as you go upstairs. Keep your back straight.

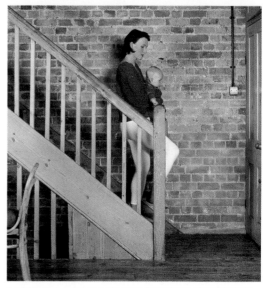

△ **3** Going down, bend your knees deeply, keeping your back straight all the time. Inhale as you lift your knee, before lowering your leg down to the next step on the out-breath.

55 Swing on the bannister

These stretches expand the movements that you make while going upstairs and downstairs. Practise them while leaning on a bannister or a table. They will strengthen your lower back and legs to walk upstairs and downstairs without strain.

◁ **1** Starting in Tadasana (28), bend your knees, back as straight as possible. Have your hands on your hips or hold on to the bannister with one hand. Go down on an out-breath, extend back up on an in-breath.

▷ **2** From the same starting point, swing your left bent knee as high as you can on an in-breath. Keep your standing leg slightly flexed. Let your leg go down to the floor as you exhale and push with your foot on an in-breath to swing your bent leg up again. Repeat a few times then change legs.

△ **3** Stand on the side of the bannister with your legs extended in a wide step, turning your back foot slightly outward. Stretch your arm on the side of your front leg, using the bannister, on an in-breath.

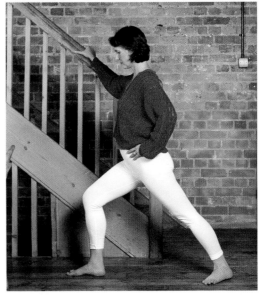

△ **4** On the out-breath, bend your knee and allow your lower back to stretch. This is an easy static version of the Walking Warrior (42). Change sides. Use any convenient support if you do not have a bannister.

Yoga with friends

It makes an interesting change to practise yoga with friends, at your home or theirs. It is always fun for mothers and babies to get together. Most babies are fascinated with other babies, so it will make your own life much easier in the future if you introduce your baby to a number of different (and friendly) people and places as early in life as possible. Your baby will build up trust and confidence through experiencing a variety of different people and faces from the earliest days.

Women who first meet during their pregnancies can become friends for life. They enjoy the fun times together and give each other mutual support through any hard and lonely times. They may also start going to yoga classes together.

There are many exercises you can do with a partner. Be inventive, yet careful. It can be very easy for the "helper" to strain the lower back. As a general rule, let the floor support the weight, rather than either partner. Friends who do yoga together will benefit from the symmetry of postures. Make sure you communicate well so that you both feel equally stretched.

56 Leg and arm stretches

This is a good routine to enjoy with a partner. Sit facing each other on a mat, a little more than a leg's length apart. Through mutual pushing and pulling of arms and then legs in symmetrical dynamic postures, you both energize and have good fun.

△ 1 Each of you bends the right knee and the right elbow, as you hold hands. Sit up straight, adjusting the distance between you until you are both in a firm sitting position with your arms at shoulder level. Now twist your upper bodies by bending/extending your arms alternately in an easy rhythm. Change legs. Breathe in the rhythm.

◁ **2** Change your hand hold, so that you are reaching to clasp your partner's opposite hand.

◁ **3** Now work your legs. Lean back on to your forearms and bring the soles of your feet against those of your partner. Keeping contact, "cycle" with your legs – forwards a few times, then backwards.

▽ **4** Finish by sitting back to back, using the pressure of your partner's back to achieve a beautiful Dandasana pose (51). Keep your feet flexed and hold the position, breathing deeply in unison. This is bonding, and your babies will feel very comfortable sharing the atmosphere that you are radiating.

gaining
strength

The feel-good factor of gentle yoga is expanded by the regular practice of movements and postures that increase new mothers' energy and enjoyment of life day by day. This is the time to replenish or renew your vitality, gaining stamina while remaining centred in mindfulness. Watch your baby copying you!

Three to six months after birth

This section continues to develop a solid foundation for long-term good posture, pelvic strength and suppleness after your pregnancy and birth. Now is the time for you to influence the state of your hips and your lower back over many years to come. With yoga, you can continue benefitting from the flexibility that the hormones of pregnancy have given you, without over-stretching too soon. The aims are to strengthen and elongate the spinal muscles in your re-aligned body.

The asanas in this section cater both for those experienced in yoga and for those new to it. You are progressively introduced to classical poses in which the hips are aligned in stretches, twists and bends with the legs open in a wide step forward. While these poses are easy if you have done yoga, you may find breathing deeply in them a new challenge. If you are new to yoga, then getting correctly into the poses as shown here will be your first step.

Once again, this time-scheme is only a general guide. You may feel more comfortable sticking with the earlier routines for a while longer. You may also prefer to take one pose at a time from this section and practise it together with earlier, already familiar poses. It is always best to proceed at your own pace, consolidating your gains and enjoying your progress.

"You are the bows from which

your children as living arrows

are sent forth."

The Prophet

57 "Easy" Warrior

This pose gives you back strong, masculine energy which you may welcome to balance the yielding and softening needed to welcome your newborn. It helps you to feel "back in your body" and makes you firm, vigorous and strong with breathing in the abdomen, solar plexus and heart combined. The Walking Warrior (42) can still be useful when your baby is awake and wanting your company. Use this standing pose to improve the walking version.

△ Stand with your legs apart and turn one foot to the side as for the "Easy" Triangle Pose (Trikonasana) (36), keeping your trunk facing the front. Breathing in deeply, bring your arms overhead with palms together in a strong lift of the upper body. Breathing naturally, improve your position. Open your chest and bring your shoulder blades closer together. Look straight ahead, keeping your chin level and your ears in line with your shoulders. Straighten your arms. When you are ready, breathe out and bend your front knee with spine erect and weight centred. Breathe in the pose for a moment, then breathe in to straighten your knee, and out to lower your arms. If you are experienced, turn your trunk forward in a Warrior Pose.

58 Triangle forward bend (Parsvottanasana)

This pose combines a stretch, a twist and a bend. The more slowly you extend and the more fully you breathe, with your awareness on the base of the spine, the greater appreciation you will get of the calm strength you gain from this pose.

◁ **1** Start in Tadasana (28). Take a step forward and turn your back foot out, keeping your weight on the back heel. Clasp both elbows behind your back.

▷ **2** Alternatively, if you can, place your hands in Namaste (10) position, between your shoulder blades, palms together, fingers pointing upwards towards your neck.

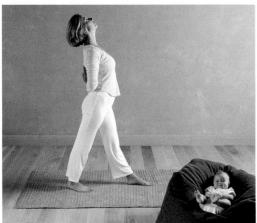

△ **3** Stretch up and back, all the way from your front foot to the top of your head, breathing in slowly and keeping your weight on your back heel. Take a few deep breaths while stretching.

△ **4** On an out-breath, hinge the spine forward from the hips and extend forward slowly, taking a few deep breaths and lifting your breastbone. When you cannot extend any further, drop your head.

◁ **5** If you are experienced in yoga, allow your forehead to rest on your front knee, keeping your weight on the back heel. If this is too difficult, loosen your arms and bring your hands forward, palms on the floor, flexing the knees if needed, to keep your back extended in the forward bend. From either position, come back up slowly, taking a few deep breaths.

Elongating the spine

As you go through successive stages of feeling aligned and stronger after giving birth, it is a pleasure to recover, or perhaps discover, the joy of stretching your spine. These deceptively simple adapted yoga poses make use of a support – a chair here – to help you enjoy the benefits of a fully stretched back. Feel the downward pull of gravity and the uplift in your lower back.

59 Leg-up sequence

This is harder than it looks! Find a support for your leg at a height that suits your physique and level of fitness – from low to high chair, to table top.

◁ **1** To begin, stand in Tadasana (28) and circle your straight arms in wide backward sweeps, lifting in the waist, breathing freely.

◁ **2** When you feel loosened up and stretched, place one leg on the chair with the knee straight and the foot flexed. Regain a balanced and upright posture and bring your palms to face each other overhead. Stretch up more on each breath out, squeezing in at the waist. Hold the position for three to five breaths. Relax your leg. Then change legs and repeat.

60 Open twist

A standing version of the sitting twist, this pose uses movement to prepare you for the classic Standing Twist (66).

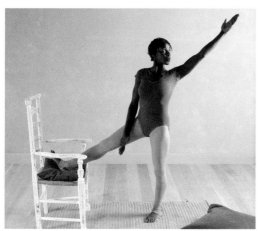

△ With your right leg on the chair, place the corresponding hand on the inner side of your thigh as a lever and twist, circling your straight arm. While opening the chest, this pose allows a stretch from the standing leg to the hand.

61 Closed twist (2)

In this twisting stretch, the pressure of the hand on the outer side of the raised leg allows a rotation of the hips.

◁ When you twist to the left this time, your leg is on the chair and the back of your right hand is the lever against the outside of your left thigh. Circle your left arm several times in wide upward and backward sweeps, lifting at the waist. Twist both sides equally.

62 Forward bend (2)

The raised leg helps you find more extension in the back as you bend forward, breathing as deeply in your lower abdomen as possible. Open the backs of the knees and enjoy aligning your hips for further stretch.

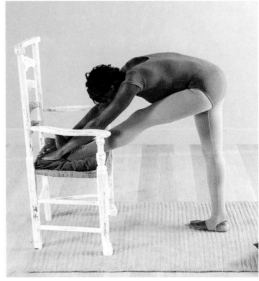

△ **1** Rest one straight leg on the chair with the foot flexed. Pull your spine up tall and raise both arms slowly overhead, palms facing each other. Stretch with the breath, then, on an out-breath, hinge forward from the hips with a straight and stretched spine. Hold the back of the chair and breathe freely.

△ **2** Alternatively, hold your foot. Keep your legs straight and make sure that your neck and head remain relaxed as you extend in the forward bend. Keep the hip of the raised leg pulled back.

63 Upper back strengthener

This exercise continues toning your central, vertical abdominal muscles as well as strengthening the upper back.

▷ Sit in an upright chair and raise your baby high above your head as you inhale. Lower the baby slowly into your lap as you exhale, remembering to use your abdominal muscles as you breathe. Repeat whenever you have a spare moment.

△ **3** To rest after these stretches, kneel down in front of the chair, with a cushion between your heels and your buttocks if you wish, and rest your folded arms on the chair seat. Breathe deeply into your back to relax.

gaining strength

Kneeling balance

As you progress in your yoga practice, make up your own routine, integrating new positions in the first basic sequences. This kneeling balance allows you to experience the full stretch which you will gain later from classic standing balances, while still remaining grounded on one hand and one knee. Balances will help you regain lightness and agility after pregnancy.

67 Cat balance

This is a wonderful stretch, which you can do after completing the Rhythmic Kneeling Sequence (47). Begin in the Cat Pose (25), kneeling on all fours with your knees directly under your hips and your hands under your shoulders.

▷ **1** With your neck and spine aligned, raise one arm and the opposite leg, making a straight line from hand to foot. Hold the position, breathing deeply, then repeat on the other side.

◁ **2** Now raise the arm and leg on the same side and stretch out straight. Hold, breathing deeply. Feel a stretch down from the hip to the foot and a stretch up from the waist to the hand, creating further space for breathing into. Repeat on the other side.

△ **3** When you have finished, lean back into the Swan Pose (24) for a moment.

△ **4** Or, bring your arms beside your body, relax in what is known as the Child Pose, breathing deeply. You may like to place a cushion under your forehead.

Shoulder stretch

The feeding of your baby is well established by now, whether you are still breastfeeding or bottle-feeding at this stage. It is time to stretch anew your arms, shoulders and neck, stimulating the flow of energy in your heart and throat Chakras. The following exercises tone the muscles that support your breasts. They stimulate the production of milk if you are breastfeeding.

68 Routine for shoulders and neck

You have already practised some of these movements separately. Do them as a sequence whenever your shoulders and neck feel tight, tense or sore. Start by loosening your shoulders and neck, sitting in Vajrasana (43): between your heels, with your big toes touching each other. If you need to, put a cushion between your heels and your buttocks.

◁ **1** Place the fingertips of one hand on your shoulder and circle your elbow several times in each direction.

▷ **2** Repeat with the other arm, then circle both elbows together. Keep your spine stretched tall and your chest open throughout.

△ **3** Now push your palms out in a kneeling version of the "Sun Wheel" Stretch (16), straightening your arms as you push away, breathing out, and bending your elbows as you bring them in, breathing in.

△ **4** Clasp your hands behind you for the Chest Expansion (45), and bring your head to the floor in front of you. Hold the position for several deep breaths, then release your hands and bring your arms beside you in the Child Pose (opposite).

Sitting poses

After giving birth, some women find that they are less flexible in the hip joints, while others feel they have gained flexibility.

Whatever is the case for you, sitting poses allow you to elongate and strengthen your spine in a variety of ways. As you stretch, bend

and twist with your legs in different positions, your "sit-bones" are your anchor on the floor and the root of your spinal stretch.

69 Seated forward bend (Paschimottanasana)

Start by sitting tall, with your legs straight in front of you in Dandasana (51), extending from your seat to your crown with your shoulders and head relaxed. Always think of extending with an in-breath before you bend on an out-breath. If you cannot bend forward without your knees coming up or your abdomen getting squashed, use a belt or a tie round your feet.

△ **1** Inhale to stretch up your spine. As you exhale, lengthen forward from the hips to reach your toes, or whichever part of your leg you can reach without strain. Keep extending the back of your knees.

△ **2** If this is comfortable, relax by bending your elbows and placing your forearms on the floor alongside your shins. Feel your hips go down on the floor as you extend your spine further with each exhalation.

70 Foot to the side forward bend (Trianga Mukhaikapada Paschimottasana) (TMP)

This is an asymmetric forward bend, so you must take greater care to sit straight. It is best to use a cushion to help you keep your weight down on the side of the straight leg. Spend more time breathing on your stiffer side to give it more stretch.

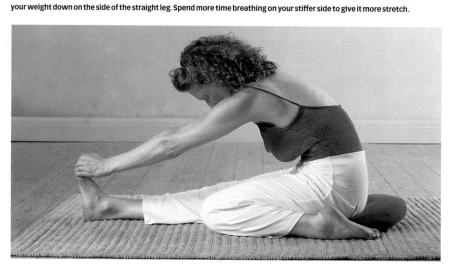

◁ Fold one leg and bring your foot beside your buttock, as in Virasana (48). Inhale and stretch your arms forward, keeping your shoulders level. Exhale and clasp your toes. Continue breathing in your lower back, extending more as you exhale. Release. Change legs and repeat.

71 "Easy" sage's pose (Marichyasana)

In this pose you are using one bent leg as a lever to further elongate the spine and release the hips. This is done first as a forward bend and then as a twist, in an easy version of the classic pose in which the bent arm entwines round the front of the knee.

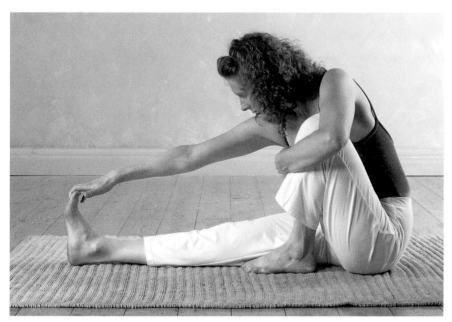

◁ **1** Bend one knee and bring your heel in against you, with your foot flat on the floor. Hold that knee close to your armpit. As you exhale, stretch forward to grasp the other foot with your free hand. If you are experienced in yoga, do the classic Marichyasana. Extend for a few breaths. Then change sides.

▷ **2** With your legs in the same position, finish this sequence with an open twist, placing your free hand on the floor behind you and stretching your spine up straight before you turn. Extend further with each out-breath, keeping your neck relaxed in the twist. Change sides.

The plough and beyond

This sequence involves positions in which your trunk is inverted, or upside down. For this reason, you should avoid it when you have a period and as long as you feel that your internal energies are involved in clearing your womb and restoring its integrity.

In this sequence, movement and rhythm help you get into the Plough Pose (Halasana) and out of it into a forward bend more easily than by holding these two poses separately. Whether you are new to yoga or have some experience, the rolling plough sequence improves your skills at the stage where you are today. Rolling is also fun as well as stimulating for both you and your growing baby. If you can't get your buttocks off the floor at first, do not worry, just laugh and try the exercise again tomorrow.

72 The rolling plough sequence

The rolling plough sequence is an unconventional, but effective way of taking your feet over your head and extending backwards before stretching forward in a forward bend, which is already familiar to you. Your rolling sequence can be as small, or as acrobatic, as you wish or can have it. Never force it. Repeating a rhythmic backwards and forwards rolling movement will get you progressively into a full Plough without strain. This is a solid foundation for a shoulder stand, which you can then move to if you are experienced in yoga or may learn as part of a yoga class later.

△ **1** Lie on the floor with your knees bent, feet flat and arms along your sides.

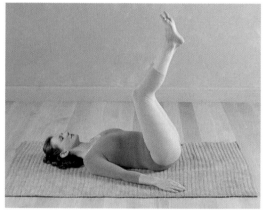

△ **2** Breathing in, lift your feet towards the ceiling, keeping your knees bent.

△ **3** Breathing out, bend your elbows and bring your hands to support your back, as you roll your hips backwards and up, bringing your knees towards your forehead. If doing this is difficult, move to 6, 7, 8.

△ **4** If 3 is easy, continue rolling your knees to your forehead. If this is as much as you can do now, use your hands to lift your hips above your head, to get your spine vertical. Take a few breaths before moving to 6, 7, 8.

◁ **5** If 4 is easy, continue your rolling movement to straighten your legs, so that your feet rest on the floor behind you, keeping your arms down beside you. Stretch on an out-breath, inhale and start rolling your spine towards the floor, bending your knees.

▷ **6** Holding the back of your knees, keep the momentum of your roll to bring you to a sitting position. If you cannot roll easily, use your hands as a support to sit up.

◁ **7** Sitting up is only a brief intermediate position in your rolling forward, extending your legs straight in front of you...

▷ **8** ...into a sitting forward bend. Stretch as you exhale and start rolling again backwards in the rolling sequence that suits you today. Get into a rhythm in which your breathing and movement allow you to roll and stretch in a relaxed way.

From relaxation to bliss

In the sequences that you have learnt and practised until now, stretching, breathing and relaxing have been equally important. You have probably become more aware of your breathing at all times, of your posture around your home and outside, with your baby and for yourself as a woman. Yoga has reminded you, in practice, how activity alternating with rest is the natural rhythm of life, as natural as breathing in and breathing out, or as day followed by night.

New mothers are often more tired from the constant attention they feel their babies need, day and night, than from lack of sleep. With relaxation, stress can be dissolved every day, as soon as it arrives. You can draw the strength you need to face unexpected challenges from reserves of deep rest. Progressively, as you become aware of your state of relaxation through regular practice of Shavasana (27), the Corpse Pose that renews you, the build-up of tension can be

averted instantly, in any position you find yourself in. You learn to "let go", to release, to just be, in a not doing, not wanting state.

At this stage, you are ready to go from relaxation to meditation, which is one of the eight limbs of yoga. In the silence and stillness of relaxation, you can experience wholeness, peace and bliss. For new

mothers, surrendering to unconditional love for their babies calls for an adequate source of self-nurture. Learning to "plug in" to the universal life-force at will in relaxation reminds us that this nurturing is infinite. "Plugging in" is simple and the more you practise it, the more rewarding it is for you, your baby and all your loved ones.

"It is vital to ask the spirits for their help or blessing, or you could wait for a long time! They never impose on us, but wait patiently to be consulted."

73 Deep rest
Every day, try to find a moment for relaxing into a deep rest. If your baby is asleep, extend your relaxation as long as you can after yoga. Being a rested mother comes top on your priority list. Bliss comes from this state of deep rest and an open heart.

△ Find a comfortable position and breathe deeply, concentrating on long breaths out. Let go and relax. Take time to return to activity.

△ Sitting up with an erect spine is the ideal
position to meditate, on the floor or on a chair.
With practice, three long breaths will take you
into this state – known in yoga as Ananda,
which means "bliss". This is the meditative
state, and the breath is the easiest tool with
which to reach this state almost instantly. After
a few more breaths, return to your external
world, bringing your inner radiance with you.
Refreshed and renewed, you can be "out there"
again, ready for your baby.

◁ If your baby is crying or
unsettled, hold him or her gently
and just be – in your heart centre,
making contact again with the
source of infinite nurturing inside
you, letting yourself be held too.

Six months onwards

From now on you can add more classical asanas to your yoga sessions, whether or not you have joined a regular yoga class for further practice. If you have not practised before, it is worth finding the school of yoga that best suits your needs as a new mother.

different "schools" of yoga

There are several traditional schools of yoga, each focusing on different aspects of this vast subject. You may need to try out several different classes and teachers before you find the right ones for you. Yoga teachers are usually quite happy to let you join their classes for a week or two before signing on.

Ashtanga Vinyasa and Iyengar yoga are very physical and demanding. Viniyoga focuses on breath with gentle movement. Energy yoga focuses on moving energy through the body using classical breathing, cleansing techniques, visualization and meditation as well as asanas. The Sivananda, Satyananda and Buddhist schools teach this more holistic type of yoga. Many yoga teachers are trained by national associations, which can put you in touch with teachers in your area.

Meanwhile, developing strength and stamina, while moving into more of the classical asanas, will give you an excellent foundation. The focus is still on poses that strengthen and "close" the pelvic and abdominal areas.

74 Tree pose (Vrkasana)

In this pose you should feel rooted, like a tree. Feel how the muscles on either side of your leg and trunk are working together, co-operating in the job of holding you upright and steady. Come out of the pose if you start to wobble. A "smaller" pose, well done, is better than wobbling in a more ambitious one! You can also stand against a wall to start with.

△ 1 Stand in Tadasana (28) and settle your breathing. Bring one foot to rest on the inner side of your other leg, take your bent knee right out to the side, pull up your spine and join your palms in Namaste (10). Breathe freely. Change legs.

△ 2 Now for the classical pose: hold one foot and bring the sole against the opposite inner thigh, with the bent knee out to the side.

△ 3 Stand up tall and raise your straight arms slowly to the sides and then overhead, palms together, breathing in. Breathe deeply and hold the pose, coming out of it as gracefully as you went in. Repeat on the other side.

75 Standing seat (Utkatasana)

This asana is like sitting on an imaginary chair. Stand in Tadasana (28) and settle your body and breathing.

◁ **1** Breathing in, raise both your arms straight up overhead. Avoid arching the lower back. Stretch right through from your heels to your fingertips, and take a few deep breaths.

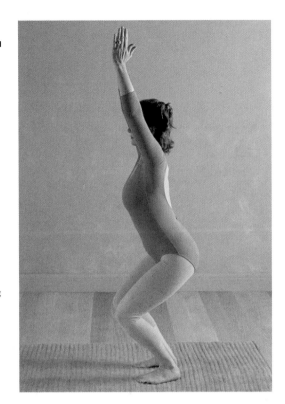

▷ **2** When you are ready, breathe out and bend your knees to "sit down", keeping your spine as nearly vertical as possible, until you are almost squatting, with your heels on the floor. Breathe deeply in the pose.

76 Standing forward bend (Padangusthasana)

This is an inverted pose, with your head lower than your heart. In contrast with the "Easy" Forward Bend (37) your feet are now together and your legs extended. Broaden the upper back and relax your head for a greater spinal stretch.

△ **1** Stand in Tadasana (28) with your feet slightly apart. As you breathe out, bend forward and hold your big toes. Improve your position by looking up as you breathe in and relaxing down even more as you breathe out.

△ **2** You can also practise the Chest Expansion exercise (as in 45 and 68, kneeling) in a standing forward bend.

Yoga for energy

As you are now following more and more the rise and fall of the flow of breath while you extend into the postures, you will be enjoying the special energy yoga brings. Rather than pushing your body to the limit in a workout, breathing in the postures as you can do them today – there is always more to come – stimulates all the systems of your physiology and increases your vital energy. Ups are not followed by downs after yoga. On the contrary, inner strength and enjoyment of life are constantly expanded.

77 Triangle pose (Trikonasana)

In this pose, the straight legs make a triangle. The back foot, firm on the floor, is your base as you stretch your spine vertebra by vertebra from the coccyx to the head, while you reach for the sky with a relaxed but straight arm.

▷ In the classical pose try to place your feet wider apart than for the "easy" version (36) – about the length of your leg – so there is more stretch. Practise first with your back to a wall, so that your head, shoulders and top hip brush against the wall as you stretch to the side and down. The point is to keep your spine elongating from the side. When you have a good "feel" for the position, practise away from the wall. Hold the position for several deep breaths, then repeat on the other side.

78 Downward-facing dog pose (Svanasana)

This is an inverted position, excellent for stretching and strengthening the whole body. The base of your spine is the apex of the pose, as you extend from the hands up your back and from your feet up your legs.

△ **1** Start in the Swan Pose (24), sitting on your heels and stretching your fingers forward. Prepare to turn your toes under.

△ **2** Breathing in, raise your buttocks into the air, coming on to your toes, and extending the back. Push your buttocks back and up, bending your knees.

◁ **3** Progressively extend your heels towards the floor, straightening your legs. Make sure you release your neck and shoulders. With each exhalation, let your back grow longer and the top of your thighs stretch. When you are ready, breathe out and place your heels on the floor and your head between your arms, so that you are looking at your navel.

79 Upward-facing dog

This phase is an upward facing stretch with the spine bending backwards while the weight is on the wrists and feet. The two phases expand the Rhythmic Kneeling Sequence (47).

▷ From the Downward-facing Dog Pose, bring your hips down without moving your toes but lifting your heels, so that your body is suspended between hands and your toes. Your head will rise. Gaze forwards and breathe deeply. When you feel strong enough, lift your hips up into the Downward-facing Dog Pose. Use the breath in these stretches: breathe out to face down and in to face up, in an easy swinging rhythm.

80 Equestrian pose

This pose continues the two phases of the Dog Pose as part of the classic Sun Salute. It is an intense toner of the legs and the hips as well as an energetic spinal stretch.

◁ **1** From the Downward-facing Dog Pose breathe in, as you swing your right foot forward between your hands. Lean hard to the side opposite your swinging leg, in order to get your chest out of the way.

△ **2** With your left knee on the floor, inhale and raise your arms above your head while dropping your hips.

△ **3** For a stronger pose, keep your back knee a short distance off the floor. Breathe deeply, then return to the Downward-facing Dog Pose on an out-breath and swing the other foot forward, breathing in. Change sides, and relax.

index